6

Duchy College

w of

sh

8-9-05

D0298897

Manson Publishing/ The Veterinary Press

Acknowledgements

First, I wish to thank Bob Condello and David O'Beirne who were instrumental in starting my work in the field of ornamental fish medicine. Marvin Lewbart, Philip Bookman, Dale Dickey, Robert Barnes, Trish Morse, Nathan Riser, Pere Alberch, William Medway, Donald Abt, Richard Wolke, Louis Leibovitz, Jack Gratzek, Ray Sis, Michael Stoskopf, Ed Noga, and Elizabeth Stone have all served as career mentors to me.

The following provided case material, illustrations, suggestions, and other assistance: Paul Barrington, Brendalynne Bradley, Michael Dykstra, Vicki Grantham, Stuart May, Jori Miller, Gayle Piner, Michael Ranucci, Gary Spodnick, Brian Tramm, Wendy Tramm, Jeff Voet, Andrea Wrangle, Todd Wenzel, Debbie Whitt-Smith, and the NCSU-CVM veterinary student body. I must also thank the helpful personnel of the NCSU-CVM Biomedical Communications Department and the NCSU-CVM Imaging Center.

I would be remiss if I did not acknowledge the fine group of contributing authors who produced the diverse and comprehensive series of cases contained within these pages. Craig Harms and Ed Noga did an excellent job of proofreading the manuscript. However, any errors or omissions are solely my responsibility.

Finally, Ray Butcher deserves special praise for his early work and effort in helping to select authors and develop the list of subjects to be covered in this text.

For full details of all Manson Publishing Ltd titles please write to:
Manson Publishing Ltd, 73 Corringham Road, London NW11 7DL.

Project management, typesetting and design: Paul Bennett
Text editing: Peter Beynon
Cover design: Patrick Daly
Colour reproduction: Tenon & Polert Colour Scanning Ltd, Hong Kong
Printed by: Grafos SA, Barcelona, Spain

Preface

Learning is a dynamic process based on experience and repetition. The text in your hands is one in a series of self-assessment guides that are designed to facilitate learning by allowing the reader to experience, via the printed page, realistic clinical situations and problems. The questions and corresponding answers in this book have been designed and selected to cover the most important and practical aspects of ornamental fish medicine. The contributors have intentionally focused on the anatomy, physiology, natural history, husbandry, diseases, and treatment of ornamental/display fish even though much of the published literature pertains to food fish species. Several questions concerning aquatic invertebrates have also been included.

This is not a comprehensive text on fish disease. Several good and recently published books adequately cover this broad subject. This self-assessment guide is designed to be a portable learning tool with state of the science images, illustrations, and information. An index has been supplied for the reader interested in selecting a particular topic and tables containing Latin names and metric conversions have been included for clarity.

As you thumb through these pages you may arrive at answers to questions which differ from those printed here. While certain questions may only have a single answer, clinical cases can be managed in a variety of ways to generate a satisfactory outcome. Consequently, an alternate solution to a problem or question may still be correct in many instances.

I encourage you to learn from these cases and questions. If you are not doing so already, please document your ornamental fish and aquatic invertebrate cases, since this rapidly developing field can greatly benefit from the accumulation and publication of knowledge on these subjects.

Gregory A. Lewbart
January 1998

Dedication
To Diane, a healer of all creatures.

Picture credits
Those mentioned below contributed photographs for use in the book (identified by question number): 13 courtesy of Brent Whitaker; 32a, b courtesy of Maryanne Tocidlowski; 37 courtesy of Betty Akiba; 44a, 46, 50, 61, 65, 187b courtesy of Todd Wenzel; 44b courtesy of William H. Wildgoose; 90a, b courtesy of Carlton Goldthwaite; 126, 160 courtesy of Tom Wellborn; 132 courtesy of Sarah Poynton; 178, 191 courtesy of Jack Gratzek; 185 courtesy of National Aquarium in Baltimore; 216a–c courtesy of Joe Spitzer. The following pictures provided by Ray Butcher have appeared in the *BSAVA Manual*: 29, 33, 52, 62, 70, 77, 81, 84, 106, 115, 121, 125, 127, 134, 143, 145, 147, 149, 151, 168, 192, 193, 204, 226, 231, 236, 249, 259. The following pictures supplied by Gregory A. Lewbart have appeared in journal articles: 7, 51, 96 in *Journal of Small Exotic Animal Medicine*; 141, 165 in *Compendium on Continuing Education for the Practicing Veterinarian*; 119 in *Journal of the AVMA*; 219 in *Journal of Fish Diseases*; 227 in *Seminars in Avian and Exotic Animal Medicine*.

Contributors

Robert S. Bakal, MS, DVM
North Carolina State University,
Raleigh, North Carolina, USA

George Blasiola, MS
Aquadine Research Corp., Healdsburg,
California, USA

Lydia Brown, BA, BVSc, PhD, FRCVS
Abbott Laboratories, Salisbury,
Wiltshire, UK

Ray Butcher, MA, VetMB, MRCVS
Wylie and Partners, Upminster,
Essex, UK

Terry Campbell, DVM, PhD
Colorado State University, Fort Collins,
Colorado, USA

Ruth Francis-Floyd, MS, DVM
Univeristy of Florida, Gainesville,
Florida, USA

John B. Gratzek, DVM, PhD
University of Georgia, Athens,
Georgia, USA

Craig Harms, DVM, Dipl ACZM
North Carolina State University,
Raleigh, North Carolina, USA

Lance Jepson, MA, VetMB, CIBiol,
MIBiol, MRCVS
University of Liverpool, Liverpool,
Merseyside, UK

Lester Khoo, VMD, PhD
Mississippi State University, Stoneville,
Mississippi, USA

Howard N. Krum, MS, VMD
New England Aquarium, Boston,
Massachusetts, USA

Gregory A. Lewbart, MS, VMD
North Carolina State University,
Raleigh, North Carolina, USA

Nancy E. Love, DVM, Dipl ACVR
North Carolina State University,
Raleigh, North Carolina, USA

Edward J. Noga, MS, DVM
North Carolina State University,
Raleigh, North Carolina, USA

Ernest Papadoyianis, MS
Exotic Reef Technologies, Boca Raton,
Florida, USA

Peter J. Southgate, BVetMed, MSc,
MRCVS
Fish Vet Group, Inverness, UK

Stephen Spina, MS
New England Aquarium, Boston,
Massachusetts, USA

M. Andrew Stamper, DVM
North Carolina State University,
Raleigh, North Carolina, USA

Michael K. Stoskopf, DVM, PhD,
Dipl ACZM
North Carolina State University,
Raleigh, North Carolina, USA

Douglas Thamm, DVM
Univerity of Wisconsin, Madison,
Wisconsin, USA

Brent Whitaker, MS, DVM
National Aquarium in Baltimore,
Baltimore, Maryland, USA

William H. Wildgoose, BVMS, CertFHP,
MRCVS
Leyton, London, UK

Roy P.E. Yanong, VMD
University of Florida, Ruskin,
Florida, USA

Common and Latin names

American oyster *Crassostrea virginica*
Angelfish (freshwater) *Pterophyllum scalare*
Atlantic seahorse *Hippocampus erectus*
Australian rainbowfish Melanotaeniidae
Balzani chichlid *Gymnogeophagus balzani*
Barracuda *Sphyraena barracuda*
Black ghost knife fish *Apteronotus albifrons*
Blacktip reef shark *Carcharhinus melanopterus*
Blue damselfish *Pomacentrus coelestis*
Blue-eyed plecostomus *Panaque suttoni*
Blue gourami *Trichogaster trichopterus*
Blue tetra *Boehlkea fredcochui*
Bonnet-head shark *Sphyrna tiburo*
Brazilian cichlid *Cichlasoma braziliensis*
Brown shark *Carcharhinus plumbeus*
Bull shark *Carcharhinus leucas*
Candy-striped shrimp *Lysmata grabhami*
Cardinal tetra *Paracheirodon axelrodi*
Channel catfish *Ictalurus punctatus*
Clown loach *Botia macracanthus*
Clown triggerfish *Balistoides conspicillum*
Cory catfish *Corydoras sp.*
Crayfish *Astacus astacus*
Damselfish *Chromis* sp.
Discus *Symphysodon discus*
Dwarf gourami *Colisa lalia*
Electric eel *Electrophorus electricus*
Emperor angelfish *Pomacanthus imperator*
Fan worm Sabellidae
Firefish *Nemateleotris magnifica*
French angelfish *Pomacanthus paru*
Golden shiner *Notemigonus crysoleucas*
Goldfish *Carassius auratus*
Gold gourami *Trichogaster trichopterus*
Gold severum *Cichlasoma severum*
Gold spot pleco *Ancistrus* sp.
Gold tetra *Hemigrammus rodwayi*
Green terror cichlid *Aequidens rivulatus*
Guitar fish *Platyrhinoids triseriata*

Horn shark *Heterodontus francisci*
Indo-pacific anemonefish *Amphiprion clarkii*
Jack Dempsey cichlid *Cichlasoma biocellatum*
Jacknife fish *Equetus lanceolatus*
Jewel cichlid *Hemichromis bimaculatus*
Koi *Cyprinus carpio*
Lemon shark *Negaprion brevirostris*
Lesser octopus *Eledone cirrhosus*
Leopard shark *Triakis semifasciatus*
Lionfish *Pterois volitans*
Mako shark *Isurus oxyrinchus*
Melon butterflyfish *Chaetodon trifasciatus*
Midas cichlid *Amphilophus citrinellus*
Moorish idol *Zanclus canescens*
Neon tetra *Paracheirodon innesi*
Nurse shark *Ginglymostoma cirratum*
Orfe *Leuciscus idus*
Oscar *Astronotus ocellatus*
Paradise fish *Macropodus opercularis*
Pearci cichlid *Cichlasoma pearci*
Pearl cichlid *Geophagus brasiliensis*
Penguin tetra *Thayeria boehlkei*
Percula clownfish *Amphiprion percula*
Pictus catfish *Pimelodus pictus*
Planehead filefish *Monacanthus hispidus*
Platy *Xiphophorus maculatus*
Porkfish *Anisotremus virginicus*
Red pacu *Colosomma brachypomum*
Redtail catfish *Phractocephalus hemiliopterus*
Rosy barb *Puntius conchonius*
Scrawled filefish *Aluterus scriptus*
Sea raven *Hemitripteris americanus*
Sheepshead *Archosargus probatocephalus*
Shovelnose catfish *Sorubim lima*
Silver dollar *Metynnis* sp.
Slippery dick *Halichoeres bivittatus*
Snakehead *Channa micropeltes*
Spiny puffer *Diodon hystrix*
Spotted raphael catfish *Agamyxis*

Common and Latin names (continued)
pectinifrons
Squirrelfish *Holocentrus rufus*
Stick catfish *Farlowella* sp.
Thick-lipped gourami *Colisa labiosa*
Tiger shark *Galeocerdo cuvieri*
Tilapia *Tilapia* sp.
Tomtate *Haemulon aurolineatum*
Whitetip reef shark *Carcharhinus longimanus*
Wreckfish *Anthias* sp.
Yellow stingray *Urolophus jamaicensis*

Broad classification of cases

Anatomy 4, 14, 20, 26, 28, 31, 32, 34, 36, 42, 43, 52, 54, 58, 59, 61, 65, 70, 71, 74, 75, 79, 84, 94, 96, 97, 98, 108, 121, 127, 140, 147, 152, 155, 156, 171, 179, 180, 199, 201, 206, 207, 209, 214, 215, 218, 221, 222, 223, 228, 235, 246, 249, 262

Anesthesia 3, 51, 63, 69, 80, 95, 110, 112, 119, 158, 213, 224, 241

Bacterial diseases 30, 41, 44, 45, 47, 53, 64, 67, 84, 92, 115, 139, 147, 169, 192, 194, 204, 226, 236, 238, 252

Fungal diseases 10, 19, 106, 107, 125, 189, 195, 252

Neoplasia 1, 3, 33, 63, 72, 77, 84, 101, 111, 123, 137, 150, 158, 159, 161, 168, 197, 213, 242

Nutrition 9, 21, 57, 103, 234

Parasitic diseases 2, 8, 13, 15, 23, 27, 29, 38, 40, 62, 69, 79, 81, 88, 89, 93, 100, 105, 109, 118, 122, 126, 131, 132, 134, 141, 144, 145, 149, 151, 160, 178, 181, 182, 183, 184, 185, 191, 193, 198, 205, 208, 212, 219, 234, 239, 243, 244, 245, 259, 261, 265

Physiology 5, 24, 36, 135, 228, 247

Quarantine 2, 43, 104, 139, 154, 176, 182, 200, 232

Surgery 3, 14, 63, 119, 158, 159, 163, 167, 172, 197, 213, 216

Therapeutics 2, 8, 11, 15, 22, 38, 41, 43, 60, 62, 80, 85, 87, 88, 91, 118, 124, 126, 129, 132, 141, 142, 146, 147, 153, 160, 181, 219, 220, 227, 233, 234, 240, 243, 244, 245, 258, 259, 263, 265

Toxicities 11, 66, 73, 82, 86, 93, 113, 117, 120, 136, 149, 162, 166, 177, 186, 190, 202, 211, 230, 256, 260

Viral diseases 39, 48, 143, 165, 176, 231, 232, 264

Water quality 6, 7, 12, 16, 17, 18, 25, 35, 37, 46, 49, 55, 56, 76, 83, 86, 91, 99, 114, 116, 117, 120, 128, 130, 133, 138, 169, 170, 173, 174, 175, 183, 187, 188, 190, 196, 202, 210, 225, 229, 230, 237, 250, 251, 254, 255, 257

Further reading

Brown, L. (1993) *Aquaculture for Veterinarians*. Pergamon Press, Oxford.
Butcher, R.L. (1992) *Manual of Ornamental Fish*. British Small Animal Veterinary Association, Gloucestershire.
Gratzek, J.B. (1992) *Aquariology: The Science of Fish Health Management*. Tetra Press, Morris Plains.
Noga, E.J. (1996) *Fish Disease: Diagnosis and Treatment*. Mosby, London.
Spotte, S. (1992) *Captive Seawater Fishes*. Lea and Febiger, New York.
Stoskopf, M.K. (1993) *Fish Medicine*. W.B. Saunders Co., Philadelphia.

1 A male *Pseudotropheus* cichlid presents with an asymmetric swelling of the frontal dome, with a bleeding ulcer measuring 3 mm in diameter. A punch biopsy, cytology, and aerobic culture of the swelling are taken (**1a** shows fish after biopsy). Aerobic culture yields no growth. An impression smear (**1b**) and histology (**1c**) of the biopsy are shown. What is your diagnosis?

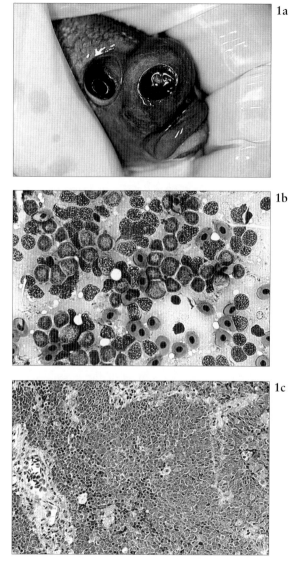

2 A hobbyist has a dedicated quarantine tank for his marine fish. He has recently purchased some fish and they have broken with *Cryptocaryon*. He asks you for recommendations regarding copper sulfate treatment.
i. How would you advise him to carry out this treatment?
ii. What are some recommendations and considerations regarding his quarantine tank?

1 Lymphosarcoma. Lymphosarcomas in northern pike and muskellunge are suspected to be of retroviral origin; a similar cause in other species has not been determined. This cichlid died before initiation of therapy. No metastases were detected.

2 i. Copper sulfate administered properly is a very effective treatment against marine ectoparasitic protozoans. Most experts in the field consider 0.15–0.25 p.p.m. as free copper ion to be the effective treatment level. A target of 0.20 p.p.m. may be the best way to ensure that levels do not fall too low to be effective or so high as to severely stress or even kill the fish. Treatment levels must be maintained for enough time to ensure that the vulnerable stage of the parasite's life cycle (the free-swimming, or tomite stage) is killed or disabled to the point of not being able to re-infect the fish. Measuring for copper levels daily with a reliable test kit is essential and additions of copper sulfate must be done as needed. If levels fall below 0.15 p.p.m., there is a chance that a fish can become re-infected. Once the parasite burrows into the fish's integument, it will not be killed by copper, and the cycle of infection may continue. The hobbyist should maintain a treatment level for at least ten days; however, 15–21-day treatments are recommended to ensure eradication of the parasite. An elevated temperature (27–29°C/81–84°F) is also recommended to accelerate parasite life cycles. This will greatly reduce the chances that parasites will be encysted during the entire treatment period and increase the probability that the tomite stage is exposed to the copper sulfate. Fish should be watched carefully for signs of copper toxicity, which may include stress coloration, diminished appetite or refusal to eat, excessive mucus production and/or respiratory distress. If fish react in such a way and it seems that the copper sulfate is the cause, water changes or removal of copper sulfate with activated carbon should be done immediately.

ii. There are many ways to set up life support for a marine fish tank, but a quarantine tank is a special consideration. Because fish will not be in these tanks for very long, lighting becomes less crucial. In fact, subdued lighting may be preferable or even critical if using light-sensitive antibiotics. Esthetic considerations regarding tank decorations should not interfere with medical treatments. For example, copper adsorbs to decorative corals or crushed coral substrates. A bare floor is recommended, except when it seems to benefit the fish to have some sort of substrate, i.e. flounders, wrasses or other fish that use substrate partially or completely to bury themselves, in which case a silica or quartz sand can be used. PVC pipe or other inert plastic items can be used as cover and hiding places for fish. Maintaining good water quality may be the single most important stress reducer for fish in a quarantine system. Careful management is required to ensure an active filter capable of maintaining proper water quality parameters when new fish are introduced to the tank. Filters must be kept active during times when the quarantine tank is not being used. This can be done artificially by using ammonium chloride to 'feed' the tank bacteria that are responsible for the metabolism and removal of ammonia and nitrites from the fish tank. Using a live fish as a permanent resident is not recommended, as this fish can act as a reservoir for parasites. Using live invertebrates is also not recommended, because many prophylactic quarantine treatments are lethal to marine invertebrates.

3 This freshwater angelfish presented because of the mass on its maxilla (3a).
i. What is the most likely diagnosis?
ii. How would you manage this problem?

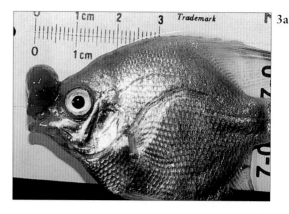

4 This is a micrograph of healthy skin from the fin of a small New World cichlid (4). Identify the black and orange structures.

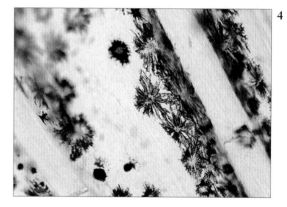

5 Occasionally, crustaceans may lose one or more limbs. How disastrous is this for the individual?

6 Half of a tropical freshwater aquarium tank has an undergravel filter. It holds a variety of fish bought from a local aquarium retailer. Areas of the tank without filtration are covered by sand. One small air stone provides air for the tank. A thermometer in the tank shows that the water temperature is 5°C (9°F) above that which is optimal for the species. No water changes have taken place since the inception of the tank, a month ago. Flaked food is offered three times a day. The fish appear sluggish and one fish has developed some dark spots on its body.
   How do you approach this problem?

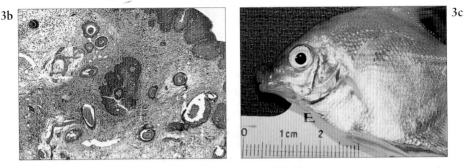

3 i. This is most likely a condition known as angelfish fibroma. It is not uncommon in this species and is believed to be associated with a retrovirus. **3b** shows the histological appearance of the tumor. Note the presence of teeth embedded in the fibrous mass. Some workers have referred to these masses as odontogenic hamartomas.
ii. Treatment involves anesthetizing the patient and debulking the mass as was done in this particular case with dramatic cosmetic improvement (**3c**). Affected fish should remain isolated from other angelfish.

4 The dark structures are melanophores and the orange structures are chromatophores. These pigment granule containing cells provide the fish with color and are under neuroendocrine control.

5 Providing the crustacean is able to avoid predation, it will regenerate the missing limbs at subsequent ecdyses (molts). Crustaceans exhibit autotomy, where as a result of trauma, or by volition, the limb is self-amputated at a predetermined weak spot. In crabs, following the loss of a limb, epidermal tissue rapidly proliferates to form a papilla, protected by an enclosing sheath. This papilla differentiates into a miniature limb with muscle, nerves, and epidermis.

In proecdysis, immediately prior to ecdysis, the epidermis begins to detach itself from the old exoskeleton, and the epidermal cells enlarge and secrete a new exoskeleton. At the same time, the previously quiescent limb papilla undergoes rapid growth so that once ecdysis is complete a new limb is formed. It may take several ecdyses for the limb to resume normal proportions.

Regeneration happens only during proecdysis. Interestingly, the loss of a critical number of limbs can initiate ecdysis, possibly by suppression of molt-inhibiting hormone (MIH) secretion.

6 Perform a water quality test. The results are likely to show raised total ammonia nitrogen, nitrite, or both. This is expected because no water changes have taken place. Lack of water changes might not be a problem if the tank is deliberately understocked. However, nitrogenous compounds will build up over a period of time, leading to poor water quality. The nitrogen cycle will have to be properly explained to the owner. A skin biopsy of the dark spots is also recommended to rule out parasites or other pathogens.

7 With regard to the freshwater aquarium tank in 6, how will you explain your diagnosis?

8 An ornamental backyard pond (1,900-L) has been stocked with 75 small goldfish (5–8 cm). During the three weeks that the fish have been in the pond, a few have died and the others are not adjusting as well as expected. Water quality parameters are good, and a large waterfall appears to be doing an adequate job of aerating the pond. The fish are observed hanging near the surface. None of the fish are eating well and rapid

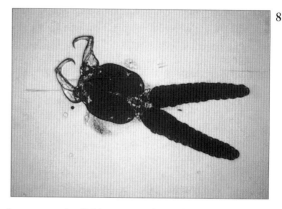

opercular movements are observed on many. A gill biopsy reveals moderate numbers of crustacean parasites (8).
i. Which parasite is this?
ii. What is an appropriate treatment strategy?

9 These captive raised Indo-pacific anemonefish (9), were cultured in a commercial fish hatchery. Occasionally, when marine fish are captive raised, or held in captivity for some time, they may experience 'stress shock' when netted, handled, or moved. Clinical signs of this syndrome include rapid, short movements followed almost immediately by total body stiffening (muscle tetanus). While mortality may reach 80%, some fish will fully recover within several hours.

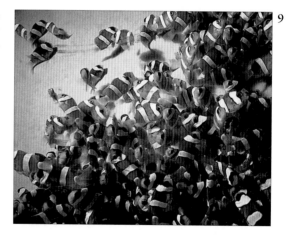

i. What is the cause of this 'stress-shock syndrome?'
ii. What factor(s) would you examine to investigate the problem?
iii. How can you confirm the diagnosis?

7–9: Answers

7 The problem of the skin lesions on one fish and the sluggishness of all the fish in the tank are indicative of poor water quality. Tests will probably show raised total ammonia nitrogen and high nitrite, with low nitrate values. These factors are a function of the nitrogen cycle. In every natural water system where animals are fed and feces are produced, there must be a balance of all nitrogen-containing compounds. This always takes the form of what is classically called the nitrogen cycle (7).

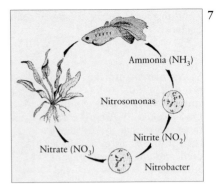

8 i. The parasite shown is *Ergasilus*, a copepod crustacean. Crustacean parasites can be identified by their paired egg sacs and antennae that have been modified for grasping. Crustacean parasites are frequently found on pond-raised as well as wild fish. Although of questionable significance when present in low numbers, they are capable of severe damage when present in large numbers.
ii. Organophosphates are frequently used to control crustacean parasites. Trichlorfon or fenthion at 0.25–0.50 p.p.m. can be applied to the pond. Because organophosphates break down rapidly as pH and temperature rise, it is important that they are applied to ponds early in the morning. Treated pond effluents should not be released into natural waterways.

9 i. Stress shock in marine fish that have been captive raised, or held in captivity for some time, is most often associated with the lack of proper assimilation of vegetable/-plant-based lipids (oils) in the diet. The substitution of soy bean meals and/or oils for the more expensive marine fish meals/oils (e.g. menhaden or herring meal, squid oil) in commercial/retail fish diets often significantly compromises the immune system over time, and results in marine fish that cannot endure the stress of handling.
ii. Thoroughly examine the long-term (15–30+ days) diet of the fish. Were they fed a diversity of frozen, live and dry commercial diets, or was their diet exclusively commercial flake food? Many aquarists substitute non-marine foods (such as lettuce for marine seaweeds) for convenience. While such substitutions are often nutritionally adequate on a short-term basis, or for intermittent feedings, a diversity of marine foods provides the optimal nutrition necessary to maintain immune system function, coloration, and growth in captivity.
iii. The dietary deficiencies described above can be clearly identified in dissections of stress-shocked fish. In both the cranial and visceral cavities, tissues will contain distinct amber-colored oil globules indicating deposition from the lack of proper assimilation of vegetable/plant-based lipids. It should be noted that most commercial hatcheries now use marine lipids exclusively in their diets to prevent such problems. Due to research into quality marine diets, captive-raised marine fish often maintain superior immune function and stress resistance compared to their wild-caught counterparts.

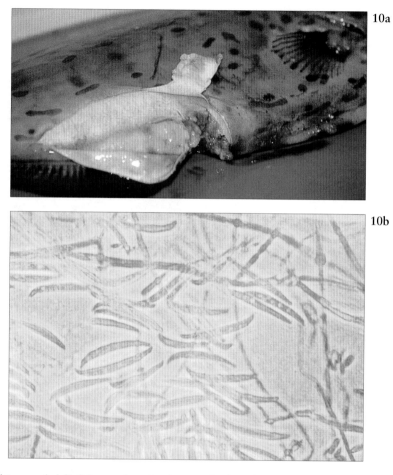

10a

10b

10 This scrawled filefish was found to be near death and was killed painlessly. It lived in a 38,000-L marine aquarium with a variety of other marine fish species. No other fish were affected and water quality parameters were within normal limits. The first figure is a gross picture of a necrotic, pale-white to yellow, friable lesion that involved a large portion of the ventral musculature of the fish (**10a**). The second figure is a microscopic view of a fungal culture that was isolated from the lesion (**10b**).
i. What is this organism?
ii. What are some of its distinguishing features?
iii. What is the clinical significance of this disease?

11 Many proprietary fish parasiticides are toxic to tropical marine invertebrates. What is the main constituent of these products that is so lethal?

10 i. *Fusarium solani.*
ii. Diagnosis is based on culturing the organism and visualizing the classic canoe-shaped or banana-shaped microconidia that are easily seen in the micrograph (**10b**). *Fusarium* cultures usually display a lavender color (**10c**).
iii. *Fusarium* infections have been reported in a number of wild and domestic animals, including humans and several species of fish. The organism is a ubiquitous opportunistic pathogen that rarely presents a problem to the uncompromised fish. Although it could not be proved, we think that this filefish sustained some type of trauma near the infected area allowing for colonization by *Fusarium*. A *Vibrio* was cultured from the kidney of this fish, indicating a bacteremia in addition to the mycosis.

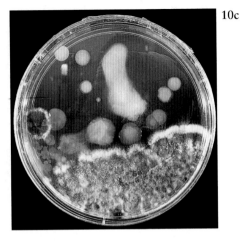
10c

11 Copper. Copper is present in these medications as the cupric ion Cu^{2+}, and in salt water much of it is incorporated into a copper chloride complex which is soluble, stable, and hence less biologically active. However, at high pH levels found in marine aquaria, copper carbonate can form, which is insoluble and will precipitate.

Dissolved copper levels greater than 0.01 p.p.m. may be toxic to a variety of invertebrates, therefore, if copper-based treatments are used in aquaria, or water is drawn from domestic water supplies with copper piping, copper levels must be monitored closely.

Copper is removed from solution primarily by adsorption to activated charcoal, or to calcium and magnesium carbonate structures. These include decorative corals and substrates, such as coral sand, crushed oyster shell, and dolomite. The rate of adsorption decreases markedly with time as binding sites are saturated. Some organisms, such as brine shrimp, bacteria, and some algae, appear selectively to take up and accumulate copper.

One of the dangers with using copper medications is that although copper is removed from solution, it is not removed from the system. A fall in pH may redissolve precipitated copper, while an increase in salinity can reverse adsorption to substrates leading to toxic levels of dissolved copper, in many cases quite some time after copper medication has ceased. Invertebrates fed on copper-accumulating organisms will suffer toxicity problems.

Copper can sometimes be eliminated from aquaria with the use of activated charcoal filtration (changed regularly) and partial water changes. Where possible, materials to which copper would adsorb or precipitate, such as coral and tufa rock, should be removed from the aquarium.

12 A client's 200-L community tank contains angelfish, cardinal tetras, hatchetfish, sailfin mollies, and several small discus. The sailfin mollies, relatively new additions to the tank, have begun shimmying (i.e. moving their fins back and forth in the same spot while their bodies move back and forth in short jerky steps while hanging in the water). The other fish look and act normally. Total ammonia and nitrite levels are zero.
i. What other parameters should you check, and why?
ii. What is wrong with the species composition of this tank?

13 A group of penguin tetras maintained in a 209-L fresh-water tank are experiencing low-level mortality. Some fish have small ulcerative lesions (2–4 mm) along the lateral body wall in the vicinity of the lateral line. A deep scraping of the affected areas reveals spherical masses embedded in the muscle tissue. Histologic examination confirms the presence of *Pleistophora* in skeletal muscle (**13**).
i. What is the treatment of choice for *Pleistophora*?
ii. What is the life cycle of the parasite?
iii. What species of fish are commonly affected?

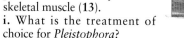
13

14 A mature female tancho kohaku koi from a 75,000-L well-maintained pond presents because the owner noticed that the fish was not eating and appeared swollen. On physical examination the skin is erythematous, the coelomic region is very enlarged, and there is a red amorphous protrusion from the vent (**14a**).
i. What conditions are on your differential list?
ii. What diagnostic tests would you perform?
iii. What is the diagnosis?
iv. How would you treat the problem?

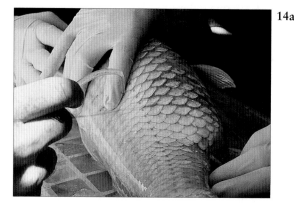
14a

12 i. The water should also be evaluated for total alkalinity, hardness, and pH.

ii. All of the fish are tropical Amazon fish except for the mollies. The Amazon fish thrive in soft, slightly acid water, whereas the mollies and other livebearers in this group prefer harder, slightly saline water.

13 i. There is no chemical treatment which is effective against *Pleistophora*. Therefore, the treatment of choice is depopulation of affected stocks.

ii. *Pleistophora* is a microsporidian parasite with a direct life cycle. These intracellular parasites are capable of reproducing by binary fission and sporogony.

iii. Although commonly referred to as 'neon tetra disease', the parasite can affect a wide range of tropical freshwater fish.

14 i. Cloacal prolapse protruding from the vent; intestinal prolapse protruding from the vent; intestinal prolapse protruding from the genital pore; ovarian prolapse protruding from the genital pore.

ii. Physical examination can yield clues as to whether the prolapse is ovarian or intestinal in origin. The ovarian tissue is usually grainy in appearance with small white to yellow follicles incorporated in the vascular ovarian tissue. Intestine will usually have a smooth surface. Cytology can further help differentiate between organs since ovarian tissue will have immature ova while the intestinal impressions yield epithelial cells and possibly fecal material.

iii. Ovarian prolapse through the genital pore.

iv. Excision of the exteriorized ovarian tissue is recommended This tissue is vascular and friable. Encircling ligatures can be placed and the distal tissue removed

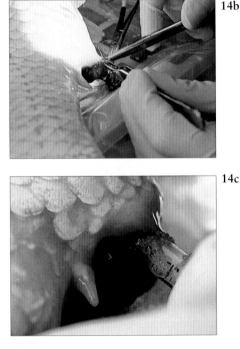

14b

14c

with a scalpel or scissors (**14b**). Depending on the fish's spawning condition, eggs can be manually stripped from the fish. To prevent further ovarian prolapse, a sterile syringe of appropriate size can be inserted into the genital pore and the eggs expressed by cranial–caudal milking pressure along the flanks to push the eggs around the syringe (**14c**). A purse-string suture can be placed around the genital pore while carefully avoiding the vent and allowing enough room for residual eggs to pass from the pore.

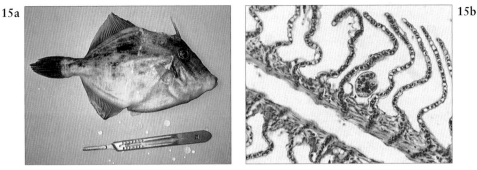

15 A planehead filefish is anorectic and severely emaciated, with multifocal white blotches on the skin (**15a**). It begins to experience equilibrium problems and is killed painlessly for diagnostic work-up to determine risk to and potential prophylactic treatment for its tankmates. A skin scraping is easily obtained (in contrast to a normal filefish with the rough and abrasive skin for which they are named), revealing several nonmotile, pear-shaped organisms of varying diameter. These organisms contain multiple small golden-yellow spherules, and have basal rhizoids. A histologic section of the same organism on the gills is shown (×250) (**15b**).
i. What is the organism?
ii. What tank treatment would you recommend?

16 A lionfish was one of several fish found dead in a quarantine facility. The fish died acutely with few premonitory signs. The only lesions observed grossly on the necropsy were air bubbles in the tissues of the fins (**16**).

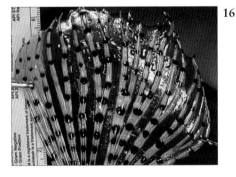

What is the most probable cause of death in this fish as well as other fish in the system?

17 What causes acid rain, and what adverse effect can it have on fish?

18 What are the recommended stocking densities for:
i. Freshwater fish.
ii. Saltwater fish.
iii. Koi and other pond fish.

15 i. *Amyloodinium ocellatum*, a parasitic dinoflagellate. Trophonts attach to gills and skin by rhizoids, causing severe tissue damage at the sites of attachment.
ii. Treatment is complicated by a life cycle that includes resistant tomonts. Copper at a free divalent ion concentration of 0.2 p.p.m. as a continuous bath is the current treatment of choice. Chloroquine has also been recommended. Treatment must continue long enough for resistant stages to form susceptible dinospores. Latent infections are common. Monitor for re-infestation following treatment.

16 Gas-bubble disease is a condition that occurs in fish as a result of supersaturation of the water with nitrogen, oxygen, or other gases. Cavitating pumps are the most common causes of supersaturation of the water. This results when air is allowed to leak into the water intake side of the pump. The condition is usually associated with pumps of 0.5 hp (about 350 W) or greater in closed systems without excessive algal growth. Diagnosis of this condition is based primarily upon the presence of gas emboli in the vessels of the fins and periorbital tissues. Microscopic air bubbles can often be found in the gills when examining fresh gill samples. Unfortunately, there is no recommended treatment, because by the time the problem is discovered, many fish have already died. Locating and correcting the pump problem will prevent this situation in the future.

17 Acid rain can occur when acidic emissions from industrial processes, car exhausts, and power stations enter the atmosphere and dissolve in the rain falling in affected areas. The acidified water can enter fish ponds directly or through water sources used to replenish ponds, it and causes a significant fall in pH. Acid water can also dissolve metals (particularly aluminum) as it travels through water courses. The acid water is irritating to the fish and can directly damage the epithelium of the skin and gills and/or cause acid-base and electrolyte imbalances. Dissolved metals can be acutely harmful to the fish. Aluminum is in its most toxic form at pH levels around 5 and it may also cause long-term damage.

A particularly dangerous period is following a thaw of accumulated acid snow, when a flush of acid water and dissolved metals may enter fish ponds and cause acute mortalities.

18 i. 1.0 cm of fish per liter of water.
ii. 0.5 cm of fish per liter of water.
iii. 15 cm of fish per square meter of surface area.
Note. Some hobbyists recommend using the figure 0.5 cm per liter for ornamental goldfish – their globoid body shape increases their average surface area per unit length when compared with most other freshwater fish (18).

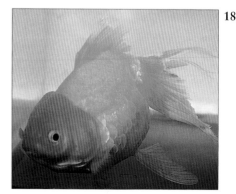

18

19 This bonnet-head shark died shortly after its removal from a 150,000-L aquarium that houses bonnet-head sharks, as well as other species of elasmobranchs (**19**). The majority of the bonnet-head sharks in the system exhibited varying degrees of similar cutaneous lesions. The other animals appeared normal. The affected sharks were lethargic and ate poorly. The bonnet-head sharks exhibited cutaneous papules, ulcerations, and erosions on the dorsal and ventral aspects of the head.

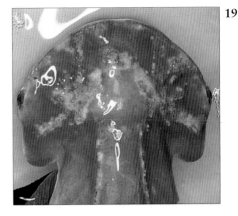

The aquarium contained artificial sea water that shared the rapid sand filtration and ozonation with a large (2,500,000-L) aquarium containing many large elasmobranchs and bony fish. The water quality parameters included temperature of 22–23°C (71.6–73.4°F); pH of 8.0–8.4; and a salinity of 32 p.p.t. The fish in the larger aquarium appeared healthy.

The gross necropsy revealed a severe liquefaction necrosis of the tissue on the head. The pattern of the lesions suggested involvement of the ampullae of Larenzini. Histopathology and cytology indicated a fungal cause. Fungal hyphae were found throughout the lesions. Microbial culture provided the definitive diagnosis of a mycosis caused by *Fusarium solani*.

How should this case be managed?

20 What are pseudobranchs (**20a**) and are they present in all species of fish?

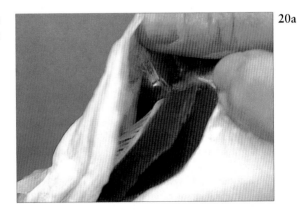

21 You need to formulate a gelatinized food diet for a group of fish to administer an oral antibiotic or parasiticide.

How would you produce such a diet?

19 Bonnet-head sharks with similar lesions failed to respond to treatment with antifungal drugs including itraconazole and ketoconazole. Because bonnet-head sharks live in slightly warmer waters than those provided in the exhibit, the aquarium temperature was raised to 24.5–25.5°C (76.1–77.9°F). After only a few months with the increased water temperature, the lesions disappeared from the affected sharks and no new cases occurred. It was concluded that water temperatures below 24.5°C (76.1°F) are immunosuppressive to bonnet-head sharks and predispose them to opportunistic pathogens, such as *Fusarium*, that are present in the aquatic environment.

20 These are gill-like structures located on the dorsal part of the inner aspect of the operculum (**20a**). They are composed of a hemibranch; that is, a gill arch with a single row of filaments each supporting secondary lamellae. Eels and silurids lack pseudobranchs. The role of the pseudobranch is unknown but it has been postulated that it is to supply well-oxygenated blood to the retina or act as a sensory structure (because of the large afferent innervation) (**20b**).

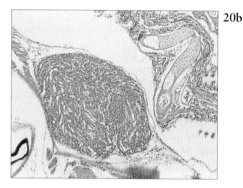
20b

21 i. The following is an example of a gelatinized food recipe. The key ingredients are the gelatin, food base, and water. Other foods and food additives can be included to meet a particular species' needs. The following ingredients make about 400 g of food.

- 70g frozen peas (thawed).
- 30 g frozen shrimp (thawed).
- 14 g (two normal packets) powdered gelatin.
- Half a tablet (adult) multivitamin supplement (optional).
- 5 ml cod liver oil (optional)
- 300 ml water.

Directions:
1 Blend the peas in a food grinder with about 25 ml water.
2 Peel the shrimp and blend them in the food grinder with about 25 ml water.
3 Mix the peas and shrimp together, pulverize the vitamin, and add to the slurry.
4 Add the cod liver oil and blend the mixture.
5 Dissolve the gelatin in 250 ml hot water.
6 Add the food mixture (with medication) to the gelatin mixture and stir well. Place the mixture in separate, convenient-to-use bags or other small containers and place in a refrigerator. After about an hour the food is ready to use, or it can be frozen until needed. Bite-size pieces of food can be provided to the fish with the aid of a cheese grater or potato peeler, especially when the food is frozen.

A popular alternative to home-made gelatin diets is a product called Aquatic Animal Gel Food which is made and distributed by Mazuri/Purina Mills Inc.

22 With regard to the diet in **21**, how would you calculate final medication concentration?

23 This is a wet mount of a fin clip from a freshwater fish (×400) (**23**).
i. Identify the parasite
ii. How would you treat this problem?

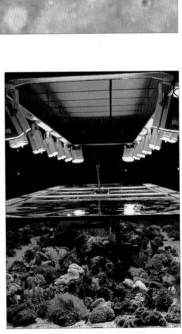

24 What are these brown–black discrete foci consisting of large, round to polyhedral cells containing intracytoplasmic pigment within their foamy cytoplasm (**24**)?

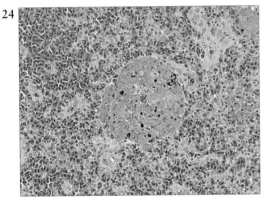

25 Lighting is regarded as being important for the well-being of a variety of invertebrates, especially corals and anemones (**25**). Why is this so?

22 The easiest way to calculate a drug concentration in food is by weight. As a general rule of thumb, many antibiotics are combined in gel food at a concentration of between 0.1 and 0.3%. For a 0.2% drug concentration, add 200 mg of drug per 100 g of food. In ideal situations, the weight of the fish will be known as well as food consumption, allowing the clinician to formulate an accurate dosing regimen.

23 i. *Ambiphrya* (formerly known as *Scyphidia*).
ii. This is an opportunistic, ectocommensal ciliate which is an indicator of poor water quality. Treatment with a formalin bath will easily kill the parasites, but improving the environment should always be part of the long-term treatment plan.

24 i. This is a melanomacrophage center (MMC), which is a normal lymphomyeloid feature of fish, found in spleen, liver, and kidney. Although MMC number and size have been loosely correlated with environmental contamination, infection, and injuries, the presence of MMCs reveals little about cause of death, and should be expected. The exact role of MMCs is uncertain, but they may represent homologs of germinal centers of mammals and birds, and are involved in antigen processing.
ii. Pigments in melanomacrophages include lipofuscin from oxidation of unsaturated fatty acids, hemosiderin from hemoglobin degradation, and melanin as a free-radical scavenger.

25 Many species of invertebrates, including the corals, anemones, and clams of the genus *Tridacna*, harbor symbiotic, intracellular, photosynthetic organisms. In the coelenterates these are algae and they are found in the gastrodermal cells of their tentacles and oral discs. Some utilize green algae (zoochlorellae), while others have golden-brown algae. These latter are often termed zooxanthellae, but they are in fact dinoflagellate protozoa of the genus *Symbiodinium*. Tridacnid clams house their zooxanthellae in mantle tissues. Certain species of sea anemones may house both green and golden-brown algae. Some sponges utilize blue-green algae.
The symbiotic algae benefit their host by releasing oxygen during photosynthesis as well as by carbon dioxide absorption. In the case of the tridacnid clams, both the zooxanthellae and their photosynthetic products are utilized through digestion by blood amoebocytic activity. These symbiotic algae have certain lighting requirements:

- Correct spectrum. The absorption peaks for chlorophyll are 400–450 nm and 600–650 nm. Water absorbs the longer wavelengths such that on a coral reef most corals are found at depths where wavelengths of 400–550 nm predominate. Therefore, lighting should be provided with strong peaks of around 425 and 650 nm to encourage photosynthesis.
- Intensity. In their native reefs, maximum photosynthetic production occurs at a depth of 10 m, where maximum light saturation in algae occurs at 35,000 lux. This means that these symbiotic algae are generally adapted to very high levels of light intensity. In aquaria, a minimum surface light intensity should be 12,000–18,000 lux.
- Photoperiod. Tropical marine invertebrates, originating in equatorial latitudes, require 12–14 hours of daylight.

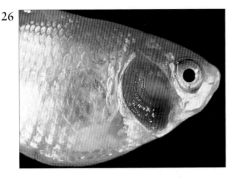

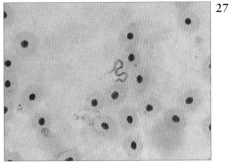

26 This goldfish died acutely of un-known causes and upon necropsy, bilateral pink masses located cranial and medial to the gill arches are noted (26). What are these structures?

27 You are working up a case of increased morbidity in some blue-eyed plecostomus and see this organism in a stained blood film (27).
i. What is this organism?
ii. What is the invertebrate vector for this parasite?
iii. What is the clinical significance of this finding, and is treatment warranted?

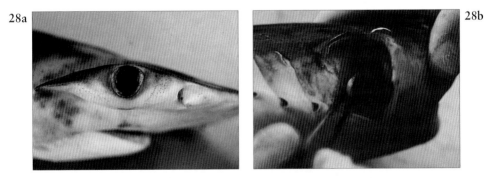

28 This recently acquired male bonnet-head shark presented dead (28a). The shark came from a 155,000-L aquarium that houses several species of elasmobranchs, including several bonnet-head sharks. Examination of the shark revealed a large hemorrhagic cutaneous lesion just caudal to the right commissure of the mouth. The shark appeared thin and probably had not eaten well. It died shortly after capture for examination. External examination of the shark revealed a large fish hook in the mouth that penetrated into the gills on the right side (28b).

How can fish hooks in recently acquired sharks be detected and, when found, how should the sharks be treated?

26 These masses are comprised of normal muscle tissue and are known as the pharyngeal pads or pharyngeal muscles. These structures help facilitate food transfer from the toothless buccal cavity to the pharynx where pharyngeal teeth grind up the ingested food.

27 i. A trypanosome.
ii. Most probably a hirudinean (leech).
iii. A large percentage of wild loricariid catfish have been found to have trypanosomes in their peripheral blood. Trypanosomes are probably part of their normal parasitic load in the wild. Laboratory studies in goldfish have shown that very high numbers of trypanosomes can cause anemia. Although hard to quantify, low numbers of circulating trypanosomes do not appear to cause significant clinical disease. There is no known treatment for this condition in fish.

28 Sharks recently captured from the wild should be closely examined for the presence of fish hooks and other foreign objects. Fish hooks are often found in the oral cavity, esophagus, and stomach. Fish hooks and other ingested foreign material can lodge in the stomach and be present in sharks that have been in captivity for many years. They have the potential to migrate into or through the stomach wall creating a coelomitis and septicemia. Fish hooks and other radiodense foreign objects can be detected by radiographic examination. Esophageal and gastric foreign objects can also be detected by endoscopy. When possible, foreign objects with the potential of harming the shark should be retrieved from the animal to prevent future complications.

Gastric foreign bodies can be retrieved from the esophagus and stomach of large sharks by inserting a large PVC pipe into the mouth. The pipe should be large enough in diameter to facilitate passage of a well-lubricated hand and arm. The pipe shields the hand and arm from contact with the sharp teeth. Obviously, proper attention to restraint of the animal is important. The shark can be restrained in a vinyl stretcher that is tied around the shark, leaving the head exposed.

Once in the stomach, the foreign object can be grasped by hand. If necessary, the stomach lining can be gathered using the fingers to bring the objects that are out of reach closer to the hand. The gastric fluids of sharks are highly irritating to human skin. It is advisable to wear protective sleeves or heavy lubrication to minimize exposure of the skin to the gastric fluids when performing this procedure. Gastric foreign objects can also be retrieved from small and large sharks using endoscopy and grasping instruments. Gastrotomy can be considered if other methods of gastric foreign body retrieval have failed and the shark is suffering from complications associated with the foreign body. In this case, the bonnet-head shark apparently died of septicemia as a result of secondary bacterial infection associated with the wound created by the fish hook in the gills.

29 An autopsy on a platy showed multiple small white nodules on the surface of the viscera of the peritoneal cavity. Low-power microscopy revealed the organism in the photograph (**29**).
i. What is it?
ii. What is the clinical significance?

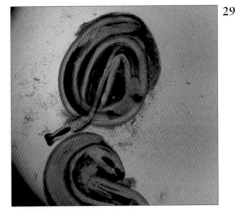

29

30 Several recently imported koi are showing extensive damage to their tails (**30**).
i. What disease is affecting the tail and peduncle of this fish?
ii. What pathogen is involved?
iii. What factors may have contributed to this problem?

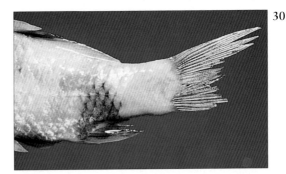

30

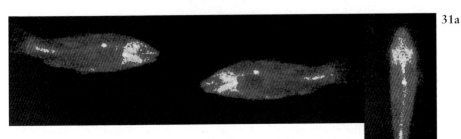

31a

31 This image (**31a**) is a nuclear scan of a five-year-old kohaku koi that presented with anorexia and strange swimming behavior. This scan was made four hours after injection of technetium-labeled methylene diphosphonate (^{99m}Tc MDP) into the caudal vein. Identify the three areas of increased activity and give the most likely explanation for why they are present.

29 **i.** The photograph shows a coiled nematode larva within a cystic structure. It is probable that this represents an intermediate stage in the nematode's indirect life cycle.
ii. This is an incidental finding and will not be a risk to other fish in the same community tank.

30 **i.** Columnaris disease (tail rot, peduncle disease).
ii. This disease is caused by infection with *Flexibacter columnaris*.
iii. Factors that predispose fish to this disease include stress from transportation, over-crowding, poor water quality, poor nutrition, underlying parasitic or fungal infection, physical injury from netting, and high bacterial loading of the water from diseased fish.

31 The kohaku koi is shown in **31b**. The three areas are: (1) The ventral aspect of the caudal spine. This area is probably caused by injection-site extra-vasation. (2) The opercular cavity. Because the gills are located here, this area is highly vascular: technetium accumulates in pooled blood. (3) The spinal column. This area of increased activity is in the area of the spine just dorsal to the swim bladder where a decreased intervertebral disc space and deviated vertebral body are radiographically evident (**31c**). The uptake of technetium may indicate inflammation and increased osteoblast activity.

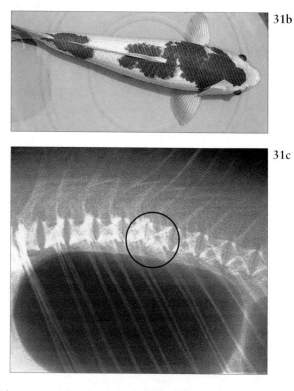

31b

31c

In this case the radiographs indicate a lesion between trunk vertebrae 5 and 6. The nuclear bone scan was performed to confirm the radiographic findings and to determine if this was an active or old lesion. The fish was treated conservatively with confinement, proper water quality, and proper nutrition. The fish recovered and regained 80% of its normal swimming ability.

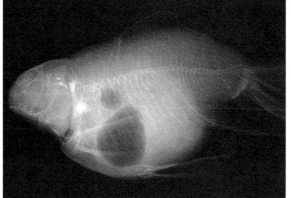

32a

32 This is a radiograph of a goldfish that was found swimming upside down at the surface (**32a**).
i. What is abnormal about this film?
ii. Is there any treatment for this condition?

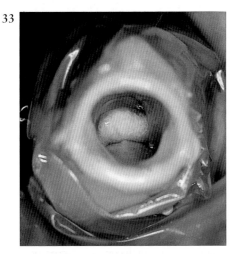

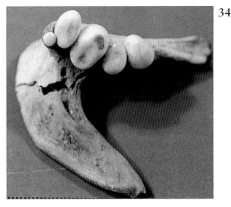

33 This koi carp presented with difficulty in eating (**33**). Examination under anesthesia revealed the lesion shown in the photograph. What is the treatment, diagnosis, and prognosis?

34 This structure was found by the side of an aquaculture pond where large carp were used to eat unwanted plants and snails (**34**).

Identify this anatomic structure.

32b

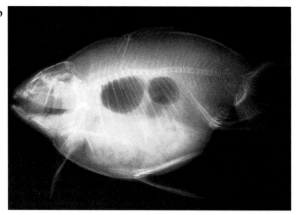

32 i. The caudal sac of the swim bladder is ventral to the anterior sac. A radiographic image of a normal goldfish swim bladder is shown here (**32b**). This fish died and at necropsy a swim-bladder torsion was diagnosed.

ii. Buoyancy disorders are very common in goldfish, especially those Asian varieties which have short, stout bodies. Some workers believe that because of these selected abnormal body conformations, the swim bladders tend to be unbalanced in these fish. Torsion of the swim bladder is not a common finding and supportive care in the form of clean water and good food is in order. Surgical correction would be an option, but such a procedure would be both risky and expensive. Aspiration of air from the caudal compartment might temporarily correct the problem.

33 This koi carp was unable to eat, although it obviously wanted to. The food was taken into the buccal cavity but then was ejected. Examination revealed a large, firm, round mass that was completely occluding the posterior buccal cavity. There was a narrow stalk that was attached to the dorsal pharyngeal wall.

The gross appearance was suggestive of a tumor. Because of the narrow area of attachment, it was felt that surgical removal was possible. This was achieved successfully with no postoperative complications.

Histopathology proved the mass to be a papilloma. The prognosis for full recovery was good in this case.

34 These are pharyngeal teeth from a large carp and are still mounted to the underlying bone. Most cyprinids have such teeth which are usually arranged bilaterally. Dentition varies between taxa. The teeth grind food against a 'carp stone', which is a thick plate at the dorsal aspect of the pharynx. The teeth pictured are several times larger than those of the average koi carp.

35 Which of the following is least likely to decrease the efficiency of a counter-current, air-driven protein skimmer (35)?
A Bubble size too large.
B Insufficient water flow.
C Insufficient air flow.
D Bubble size too small.

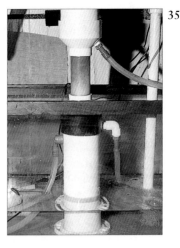

36 This is a lateral radiographic view of a Midas cichlid (36).
i. Is the radiolucent swim bladder normal?
ii. How do cichlids and many fish with spiny fin rays regulate gas in the swim bladder?

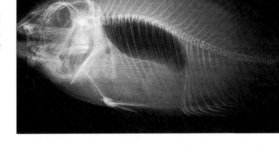

37 A pond owner wants to know if she should purchase a de-icer. In her geographical area, the temperature is below freezing for an average of 18 days per season. What advice can you offer?

38 A hobbyist's prize fish is covered with white spots. The fish is removed from the tank and *Cryptocaryon irritans* is identified by making a wet mount from a skin scraping. There are only two other fish in the tank, neither of which exhibits any signs of infection. The hobbyist has no hospital tank.
i. How would you treat the affected fish?
ii. Would it be necessary to treat the other fish?

35 D. An extremely fine mist of bubbles is needed efficiently to extract dissolved organic material from the water. The air flow should be adequate to make the entire skimmer column milky white, and the usual recommendation is for a water pump capable of turning over the entire tank volume once per hour.

36 i. This is a normal swim bladder. Careful inspection of the radiograph will reveal a thin septum located in the caudal aspect of the swim bladder. This is normal for the Midas cichlid and related species.
ii. Cichlids and many fish with spiny fin rays are physoclistous, i.e. they regulate gases in the swim bladder by a rete mirabile, which allows for vascular diffusion of gases. Most adult physoclistous fish do not have a patent pneumatic duct, a tube which connects the esophagus and swim bladder.

37 Brief periods of icing are not harmful to pond fish if the pond is of sufficient depth (a section of the pond should have a depth of at least 120 cm). In a location where the pond is frozen for a majority of the winter (**37**), a de-icer may be necessary to provide a water–air interface for gas exchange. If an external filtration system is run throughout the winter, this may agitate a section of the water surface enough to prevent icing, and the filter itself will facilitate gas exchange.

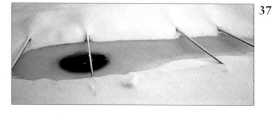
37

38 i. Two common treatments are the freshwater dip and the formalin dip. Fresh tap water can be used, taking care to dechlorinate with sodium thiosulfate. Adjust the temperature and pH using common baking soda so that it matches the marine tank. The freshwater dip should be done for at least three minutes to allow the freshwater to penetrate the fish's mucus layer and osmotically enter the protozoan, causing the cell to rupture. If the fish seems to be tolerating the dip, it can be extended to four or five minutes.

A formalin dip can be prepared using water from the marine tank. Formaldehyde (37%) is added at 100 p.p.m. or approximately 1 ml per US gallon. The fish is bathed in this solution for an hour. *Warning!* Many juvenile and scaleless fish are sensitive to formalin, as are all elasmobranchs. Should the fish exhibit distress during the dip, discontinue immediately and move the fish to recovery water from the tank.

Treating an individual fish in the above manner may kill most of the adult parasites, but it will not harm the encysted stage of this protozoan. A long-term treatment (i.e. copper sulfate) is necessary to ensure eradication of the problem.
ii. Although the other fish in the tank do not exhibit signs of disease, the entire tank (including the affected fish) must be treated for this parasite. As previously stated, a long-term treatment that would last through all stages of the parasite's life-cycle would provide the best success.

39 i. What is the cause of these lesions, which resemble molten candlewax, on the dorsal fin of this koi (**39**)?
ii. How can this disease be controlled?

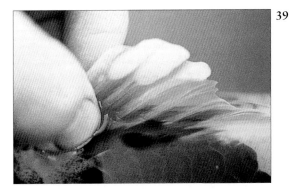

40 This crayfish has numerous raised nodules on its carapace and head (**40**).
i. What is the cause of this condition?
ii. What is the treatment?

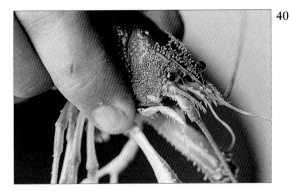

41 Skin ulceration in koi is a common problem (**41**).
i. What are the causative agents of these ulcers?
ii. Describe how you would treat these lesions?

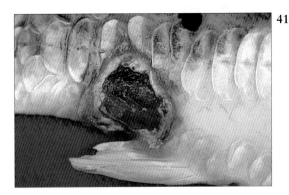

42 Where would you give an intraperitoneal injection to a fish?

39 i. Carp pox, caused by infection with *Herpesvirus cyprini*, also called cyprinid herpesvirus 1 (CHV1). These lesions are often classified as neoplasia but are basically an epidermal hyperplasia.
ii. The disease is often seasonal and usually affects only a few fish in the pond. Lesions develop in low water temperatures (winter/spring) and regress when water temperatures increase. Treatment is seldom required because the disease is rarely fatal and is usually self-limiting. Lesions may recur the following year.

40 i. These are the eggs of another aquatic invertebrate, most likely an insect. This is a common condition of freshwater crayfish and does not appear to affect the animal.
ii. This condition does not require treatment because the eggs will disappear after they hatch or the eggs and other attached materials will be shed when the crayfish molts.

41 i. Infection with *Pseudomonas* and *Aeromonas* bacteria, particularly *Aeromonas hydrophila* and atypical *Aeromonas salmonicida*.
ii. Treatment often depends on the severity of the lesions but usually requires general anesthesia and local debridement. This should be followed by topical application of antiseptic/antibiotic and a protective waterproof paste. Improved water conditions with the addition of salt at 2–3 p.p.t. (2–3 g/L) and raising the water temperature often improves recovery. The use of systemic antibiotics by injection and/or inclusion into the feed is often required.

42 In the caudal ventral abdomen with the fish held so the viscera fall away from the injection site. The needle is carefully inserted between the scales at about a 45° angle. A showa koi receiving an intraperitoneal injection is shown (**42**).

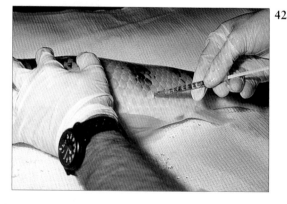

42

43 The owner of a synodontid (upside down) catfish contacts you because the fish's left eye appears cloudy (**43**). You examine the fish and note that the affected eye is indeed cloudy and possibly ulcerated. The fish is in a quarantine tank with several other fish and some driftwood and a sponge filter. The right eye appears normal.
i. What is at the top of your differential list?
ii. How would you confirm the diagnosis?
iii. How would you manage this problem?

44 A tank of platys at a local wholesaler have begun to experience mortalities (**44a**). Many of the fish hang listless in the water near the surface. A few seem to have a white ring around their mouth, and/or whitened areas on their back and along the borders of their fins. Some of these areas are hemorrhagic.

What do you suspect is the problem?

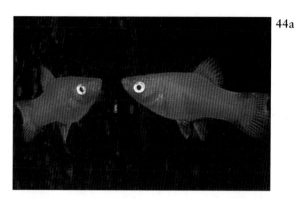

44a

45 Soft corals and anemones require delicate handling, and, in the case of the latter, are often best moved while still attached to a suitable piece of rock or substrate (**45**). Why is this?

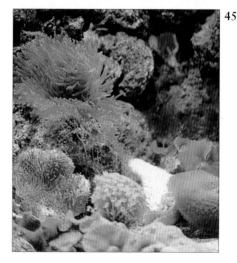

45

46 Of activated carbon or zeolite, which one's activity can be restored? How is this accomplished?

43 i. Corneal ulcer or abrasion
ii. Fluorescein staining of the eye. In this case, the eye retained the stain after flushing, confirming a significant corneal defect (43).
iii. There are two ways to manage this condition. If the fish is easy to catch and owner compliance is adequate, topical antibacterial ophthalmic ointment can be applied directly to the eye two to four times daily. The ointment should be allowed to remain on the eye for at least 60 seconds before returning the fish to the aquarium.

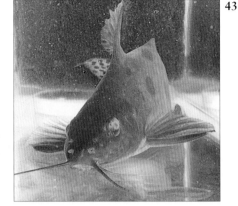
43

If this course is not practical, a broad-spectrum antibiotic can be added to the water in a hospital aquarium and the fish treated for five to seven days or until the cornea heals. This fish responded well to daily, five-hour bath treatments of 20 p.p.m. nitrofurazone.

44 Skin and fin biopsies confirm the presence of columnaris disease (*Flexibacter columnaris*). The 'haystack' appearance of the bacteria is characteristic of this organism (44b).

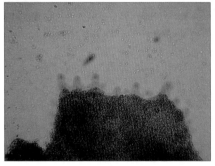
44b

45 Soft corals and anemones are particularly susceptible to trauma, which is often followed by secondary bacterial infection. *Vibrio* spp. are frequent isolates from lesions in a variety of invertebrates, including mantle ulcers on the lesser octopus. In comparison with commercially farmed invertebrates, bacterial and other diseases have not been investigated to any great extent in the majority of marine invertebrates encountered in the aquarium trade. Antibiotic therapy is therefore largely empirical, with dose rates based on anecdotal regimes rather than pharmacokinetic studies.

46 Zeolite's activity can be restored by immersion in a 1.0% sodium chloride solution (46). Activated carbon must be replaced every four to eight weeks, depending on the biological load and filtration rate.

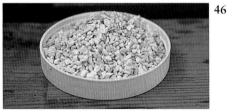
46

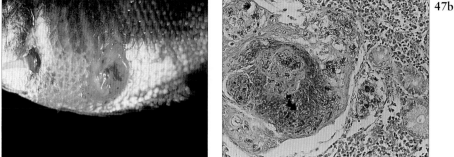

47a
47b

47 This ulcerative lesion developed in a dwarf gourami that had not been eating well and was slightly emaciated (**47a**). Histopathology revealed numerous dermal and visceral granulomata (**47b**). What is your diagnosis, and how can you confirm it?

48 A cutaneous lesion was observed on the body of a jackknife fish that was being held in a salt water quarantine tank. The lesion had a raised, gray, cauliflower-like appearance. The fish was eating and exhibited normal behavior. The water quality parameters were within normal limits and the other jackknife fish in the aquarium appeared normal. A small biopsy of the lesion was obtained and examined directly under the microscope.

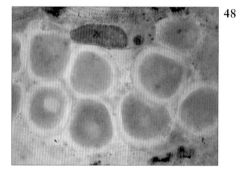

48

i. What is the diagnosis of the lesion based on this photomicrograph (×10 obj) (**48**)?

ii. How would you treat this fish?

49 An owner reports that the fish in her previously stable aquarium are spending a majority of time at the surface of the water and appear to be trying to gulp air.
   What is the most likely problem?

50 You look into one of your client' tanks of South American fish and notice the following: the silver hatchets and one small silver arowana are hanging near the surface; the black ghost knives are lying on their sides on the bottom of the tank; and the spotted raphaels, gold spot plecos, and gold tetras are swimming slowly in the middle of the water column. Which fish should you worry about?

47 With a history of wasting and debilitation, an important differential to consider, especially in pet fish, is mycobacteriosis. An acid-fast stain can help support the diagnosis, but culture on specific media like Loweinstein–Jensen agar and identification are required for definitive diagnosis. Besides *Mycobacterium*, other acid-fast bacteria like *Nocardia* have also been reported in fish. Most of the mycobacteria isolated from fish are atypical, with *Mycobacterium fortuitum* and *Mycobacterium marinum* being the most common.

48 i. Based upon microscopic examination of the excised tissue, the dermal cells (fibroblasts) appear greatly enlarged. This is indicative of lymphocystis disease. Other conditions that are associated with gross lesions that resemble those of lymphocystis include: chlamydial epitheliomas, clusters of trematode cysts, and dermal sarcomas. Cytology and histopathology are helpful in the differentiation of these disorders. The photomicrograph of the lymphocystis lesion also includes a trematode.
ii. Lymphocystis is caused by an iridovirus. The disease is typically self-limiting and lesions will disappear within a few weeks. Although the type of transmission is unknown, it is speculated that the disease is transmitted by direct contact. Therefore, affected fish should be isolated from other fish until the lesions have disappeared to prevent spread of the disease.

49 Decreased dissolved oxygen is the most common reason for fish displaying this behavior. The most common cause is an increase in water temperature, caused by an improperly set or malfunctioning heater thermostat. Fish will spend a majority of the time at the surface where the oxygen tension is nominally higher.

A similar problem can occur during long periods of high ambient temperature in nonclimate-controlled rooms. The temperature in the aquarium can rise to dangerous levels due strictly to heat conduction from the surrounding air. A malfunctional aquarium heater can also cause this problem, or worse yet, kill fish with extremely high temperatures. Aquarists should be advised to purchase top quality submersible aquarium heaters.

50 The gold spot plecos (50) and spotted raphael catfish, since they normally occupy the substratum of the aquarium.

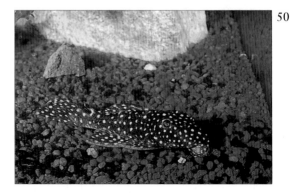

50

51 Describe how you would obtain a useful fecal sample from a fish.

52 What abnormal clinical sign is shown in the photograph (52), and what other signs are often associated with this problem?

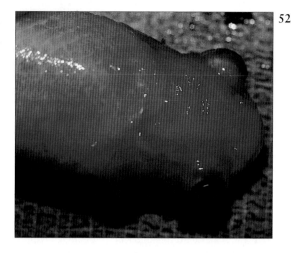

53

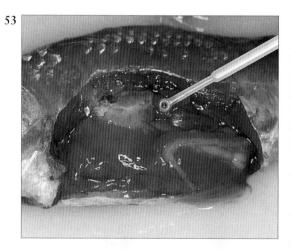

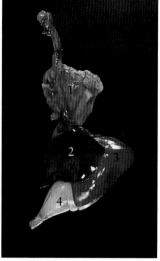

53 Bacteriologic samples are frequently taken from the kidney when examining fish (53).
What are the reasons for this?

54 Identify the four chambers of a fish heart (54), and how do they differ histologically?

51 Fecal samples can yield valuable diagnostic information, but if taken from the bottom of an aquarium or pond, they are frequently contaminated with saprophytes and other nonpathogenic organisms. It is also hard to identify the fish that produced the feces with this technique. The best

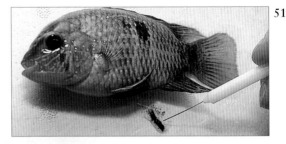

method involves isolating the fish in a clean bucket or bag until a sample is produced (usually overnight). A second technique involves tranquilizing the fish with tricaine methane sulfonate. Tranquilized fish like this green terror commonly defecate (51).

52 This photograph is of a goldfish showing bilateral exophthalmos (popeye). This condition is generally the result of retrobulbar edema and fluid retention. The fluid can also accumulate elsewhere and other signs that may be seen include edema of the vent and skin and gross distension of the abdomen. The latter can become so marked that the scales tend to stand out at an angle giving the fish a 'pine cone' appearance.

Other causes of exophthalmos include ammonia toxicity, neoplasia, gas bubble disease, trauma, bacterial disease, and ocular parasites.

53 Bacterial septicemias are common in fish. The kidney is a major filtering organ and any systemic bacterial infection should be found here. The kidney can usually be exposed aseptically by carefully displacing the abdominal organs and swim bladder, allowing a bacteriological loop or swab to be conveniently and easily inserted. Bacteriologic samples are occasionally obtained from external lesions, particularly if it is not intended to sacrifice the fish under examination. These are frequently contaminated with insignificant environmental organisms, however, and care must be exercised in the interpretation of results.

54 The four chambers are: the sinus venosus (1), atrium (2), ventricle (3), and the bulbus arteriosus (also referred to as the conus) (4). The wall of the sinus venosus is very thin and is almost completely devoid of cardiac muscle. It consists of an epicardium and an inner layer of endothelium, the endocardium. Few isolated cardiomyocytes and little melanin are present between the epicardium and endocardium. The atrium is anterior to the sinus venosus. This thin-walled chamber is thicker than the sinus venosus and consists of cardiac muscle covered by epicardium and an inner portion of endothelium-lined cardiomyocytes, arranged in a widely spaced network bathed by blood. The ventricle is the most muscular chamber, consisting of an outer compact layer and a thicker, inner, spongy layer of anastomosing cardiomyocytes lined by endothelium. The outer layer is supplied by the coronary vessel and is lined on the outer surface by epicardium. The bulbus arteriosus lacks cardiac muscle and is composed of elastic connective tissue and smooth muscle.

55 Some sailfin mollies (55), cory catfish, and small characins (tetras) have been placed in the same aquarium. The water quality parameters are within normal limits and the water is soft and acidic.

Which fish will not thrive, and why?

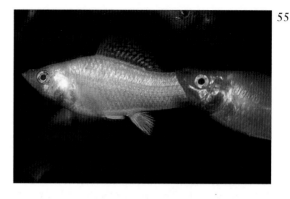

56 What is the most common cause of water quality problems when using an external canister filter (56)?
A Improper choice of filter media.
B Improper positioning of water inlet and return tubes.
C Too infrequent cleaning.
D Improper arrangement of filter media in the canister.

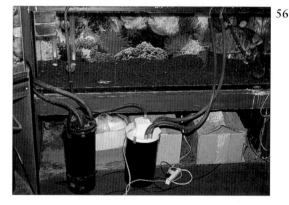

57 Which of the following fish are most likely to consume live aquatic plants?
A Rosy barb.
B Pimelodid (pictus) catfish.
C Freshwater angelfish.
D Black tetra.

58 What is the difference between the blood flow of mammals and fish?

59 What is the normal histologic organization of the trunk kidney?

55 This question has been included to emphasize the fact that what is normal for one species is not normal for another. It is very important that homework is done before fish are stocked. Once the optimal water quality is known for each species, care must be taken to ensure that compatible species are placed in the same tank. The live-bearing mollies will not thrive in soft acid water. Remember also that water plants have preferred ranges for water quality. If water is too soft and acid, many plants will not thrive.

56 C. Because of the high flow rate associated with most canister filters, large amounts of filtered debris can accumulate very quickly. This mechanically disrupts the flow of water through the filter, decreasing efficiency, and allows toxic compounds to be released during the decomposition of the debris.

Many high-flow canister filters need to be changed as frequently as once per week. More frequent changes may be necessary if using diatomaceous earth, as its small pore size predisposes to faster clogging.

57 D. Black tetra. Although many species may consume plant material or damage plants by consuming organisms living on their leaves, characins as a group are most likely to consume live plants to an unacceptable degree.

Plants are also at risk in tanks containing large cichlids, which tend to disturb the gravel in which the plants are rooted.

58 Fish have a single-pass system. Deoxygenated venous blood is received by the heart and pumped to the gills to be reoxygenated and then distributed to the rest of the body before returning to the heart. Mammals have a double-pass system with deoxygenated blood being received by the right atrium and pumped by the right ventricle to the lungs for oxygenation. The reoxygenated blood returns to the left atrium and is redistributed to the body by the left ventricle.

59 The piscine kidney is not separated into the medulla and cortex as in the mammalian kidney. The trunk kidney is composed of identical nephrons (which are the functional excretory units of the kidney) mildly separated by small amounts of hematopoietic elements (59).

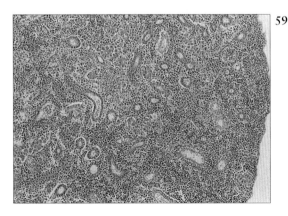
59

60 i. What is the likely cause of this fish's buoyancy problem (**60a**)?
ii. How would you confirm your diagnosis?
iii. How might you treat this condition?

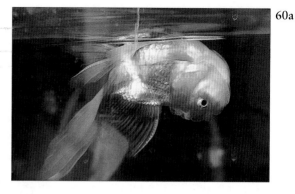

60a

61 One fish of a group of eight Lake Victoria cichlids in a 150-L aquarium has stopped eating, is staying away from the others, and appears to have an enlarged but closed buccal cavity (**61**). The other seven fish appear unaffected. What is your primary rule-out?

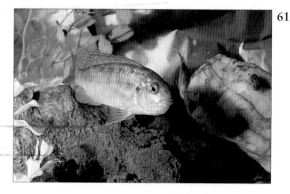

61

62 i. Identify the parasites seen within the small intestine in the photograph (**62**).
ii. How are they often observed in the live fish?
iii. What treatment would you recommend?

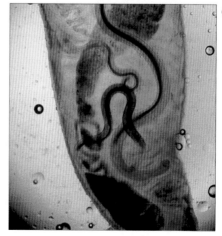

62

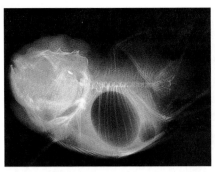

60b

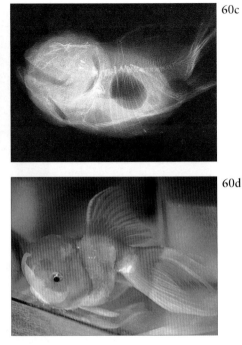

60c

60d

60 i. An abnormally inflated swim bladder.

ii. Radiography (**60b**).

iii. Aspiration of air from the overfilled compartment. The second radiograph and gross picture were taken after 3.0 cm³ of air was removed from the swim bladder (**60c**). After this procedure, which was performed with a 25-gauge needle, the fish became negatively buoyant but was able to eat and appeared to be more comfortable (**60d**). This is a common disorder of Asian fancy goldfish and is frequently difficult to resolve. Because the swim bladder has a patent connection to the esophagus by the pneumatic duct in goldfish and other cyprinids, it is theorized that there may be a nutritional component to the problem. Another theory rests on the fact that many of these varieties of goldfish have been bred for abnormal conformation and thus are prone to be 'off balance.' Anecdotal reports of fish improving after being fed fresh or cooked peas have been confirmed by the author, although no controlled studies have been performed regarding this 'treatment.'

61 These fish are mouth brooders and the 'affected' fish is likely a female with eggs or young in the buccal cavity.

62 i. The photograph shows adult nematode worms of the genus *Camallanus* in the intestine of a platy.

ii. These red worms may be up to 1 cm in length and are more common in live-bearing tropical fish, where they may be seen protruding from the vent. Infestation may result in weight loss and ulceration of the gut.

iii. Treatment is often successful using anthelmintics (e.g. levamisole) in the water.

63 This freckled grouper, approximately 82 cm in length, presented with what was described by the aquarist as a papillomatous growth around its vent. The animal was housed in a 2,500,000-L aquarium with 36 large elasmobranchs and numerous bony fish. The water quality parameters included a temperature of 24.5–25.5°C (76.1–77.9°F); pH of 8.0–8.4; and salinity of 30–32 p.p.t. The artificial sea water is treated with rapid sand filtration and ozonation. The aquarium fish are fed whole or cut fish.

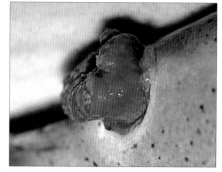

The fish was netted from the exhibit for examination.
i. What are the possible causes for the lesion (63a)?
ii. How would you examine this fish, and what steps would you take to obtain a diagnosis and implement treatment?

64 This mature black tetra presented for an erosive lesion of the maxilla and mandible (64). The owner noticed the lesion several weeks ago and it has progressed to the point that the fish has difficulty eating.

What problems are on your differential list?

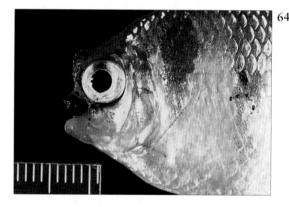

65 A client complains that her fish has developed a fungal infection on the ventral fin in front of the tail (65). She tells you that several distinct white spots have developed over the past several months, leading her to this conclusion. Otherwise the fish and its tankmates are normal. What is the explanation?

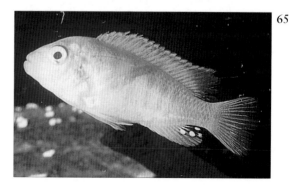

63 **i.** The gross appearance of the lesion resembles papillomatosis, which could have an inflammatory etiology, or the lesion could be a papillomatous neoplasia. Chronic inflammatory diseases caused by a variety of pathogenic organisms (i.e. bacterial, parasitic, and possibly mycotic) of the lower intestinal tract could result in the formation of such a lesion.

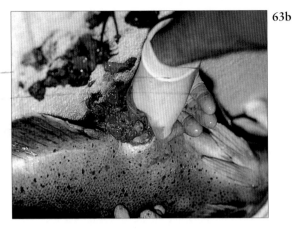

63b

ii. A fish of this size should be examined under general anesthesia. A biopsy of the tissue for histologic examination may be helpful in determining the cause of the lesion. The grouper was anesthetized using 100 p.p.m. tricaine methanesulfonate (MS-222). A physical examination revealed a chronic prolapse of the distal colon. Further examination of the lower intestinal tract revealed an impaction resulting from partially digested fish (**63b**). This material was removed using sponge forceps and flushing with warm saline. Following removal of the impacted material, the necrotic prolapsed tissue was excised and the healthy tissue was sutured to the vent using simple interrupted 2-0 EU sutures. The excised tissue was submitted for histologic examination. Recovery from the anesthesia was uneventful and the fish was returned to the exhibit after three weeks. The histopathology indicated a chronic inflammatory response to the lower intestine. No etiologic agent could be determined.

64 Neoplasia and mycobacteriosis. Biopsy and subsequent histologic examination confirmed this to be a case of mycobacteriosis. Because of the severity of the lesion, the fish was humanely destroyed.

65 This condition is normal. The males of many species of African cichlids possess decoy egg spots on their anal fins. During courtship, the female deposits her eggs in the nest while the male fertilizes them. Shortly after the eggs are deposited, the female retrieves the eggs and holds them in her mouth. In her attempt to retrieve the male's 'decoy eggs,' she inhales sperm, increasing fertilization efficiency. The number of egg spots varies between species and there is also individual variation.

66 One of your koi-owning clients contacts you early one morning and she is very distressed. All nine of her prized koi are dead and floating in the pond (66). They were apparently normal last night and had good appetites for their evening feeding. The 2,500-L pond is supplied with city water and has adequate biological and mechanical filtration as well as an aerating fountain. All components are functioning normally but the owner mentions that the person who 'topped off' the pond last night with water had inadvertently left the hose running all night (the hose can be seen in the photograph).

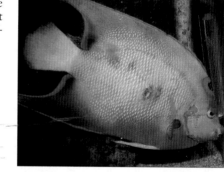

i. What is at the top of your differential list?
ii. How can you confirm your diagnosis?
iii. What are the principles of chlorine toxicity?
iv. What other conditions resemble chlorine toxicity?
v. How can such a problem be prevented in the future?

67 This queen angelfish has multiple ulcerative lesions on its body (67). What problem would be at the top of your differential list?

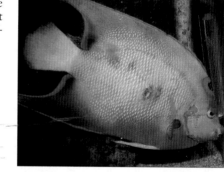

68 i. What is the translucent duct indicated in this goldfish (68)?
ii. What is its purpose?

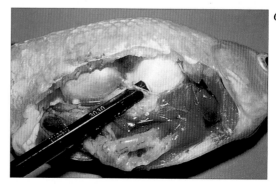

66 i. Chlorine/chloramine toxicity
ii. By testing the water for chlorine levels. In this particular case, levels were recorded at 1.2 p.p.m. (several hours after the water sample was obtained). A bench-top chlorine titrimeter was used, although much simpler and less expensive colormetric tests are available.
iii. Chlorine reacts with living tissues causing acute necrosis. Because the gills are vulnerable and exposed directly to the aquatic environment, this can lead to respiratory difficulty and asphyxiation. Fish experiencing chlorine toxicity will appear very stressed. Morbidity and mortality depends on chlorine levels in the water. High levels (greater than 1.0 p.p.m.) may cause fish to succumb in hours or even minutes. Affected fish may be piping at the surface, swimming abnormally, and they may appear pale and mucus covered. Most municipal water has been chlorinated to disinfect it for safe human consumption. Although relatively harmless to humans, chlorine can be deadly to fish. The amount of chlorine in tap water may fluctuate but is usually between 0.5 and 2.0 p.p.m. Chlorine can be 'bubbled' out of water by aerating for several days in a container with a large surface area. Another commonly used disinfectant is chloramine. This compound combines chlorine with ammonia, both of which are harmful to ornamental fish. Unlike chlorine, chloramine does not produce trihalomethanes, which are toxic to humans.
iv. Many toxic conditions will resemble chlorine poisoning (ammonia, copper, and organophosphates). An accurate history will usually rule these out. Hypoxia caused by overcrowding or poor aeration can also look like chlorine toxicity.
v. In cases where the fish are still alive, the contaminated water must be immediately neutralized or the fish removed to clean, chlorine-free water. A number of commercially available compounds quickly and safely remove chlorine from water. These products usually contain sodium thiosulfate, which inactivates chlorine through a chemical reaction in which sodium chloride is formed. Sodium thiosulfate is inexpensive, effective, and safe (just 7 g of sodium thiosulfate will remove the chlorine from 1,000 L of municipal water with chlorine concentrations as high as 2.0 p.p.m.).

After the chlorine has been removed, the water containing the fish should be aerated well with room air or preferably 100% oxygen. Temperate species like goldfish and koi will benefit from reducing the water temperature to increase dissolved oxygen levels. When possible or practical, administering dexamethasone intravenously or intraperitoneally at a dose of 2.0 mg/kg every 12 hours may improve the prognosis.

67 Ulcerative bacterial disease. Culture and biopsy of these lesions confirmed this as a case of ulcerative mycobacteriosis. Generally considered to be untreatable, there are empirical accounts of a number of fish improving on long-term oral or injectable antibiotic therapy.

68 i. This is the pneumatic duct.
ii. This duct connects the swim bladder to the esophagus and maintains an active communication, allowing the fish to regulate its buoyancy.

69 This is the trunk of a large sanke koi (69a). The fish had recently been lost from its pond following a severe hurricane and was located eight days later swimming in a stream about a kilometer from the owner's property. When the pond flooded, the fish found its way to a stream and then swam into a larger stream where a woman noticed some teenagers throwing stones at the fish. The

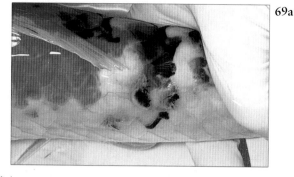

owner was contacted and the fish swam into a net. Several weeks later the owner noticed a number of green, raised lesions on various parts of the fish's body. The lesions ranged from 3–10 mm in diameter and were red at the margins.
i. What would be your diagnostic plan?
ii. How would you treat this condition?

70 i. What abnormal sign is shown in the photograph (70)?
ii. What other signs are often associated with this problem?

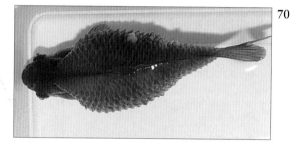

71 What is this organ (71)?

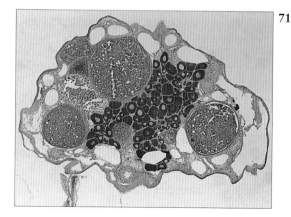

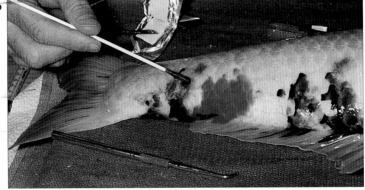

69 i. Test the water and biopsy the lesions. Water quality parameters were unremarkable. Biopsies of the lesions revealed a mixed green and blue–green algal infection. Samples were saved for culture and histology.

ii. Algal dermatitis has been reported in fish but does not appear to be common in koi. In this case, the fish was anesthetized with tricaine methanesulfonate (MS-222) (150 p.p.m.) and the wounds were carefully debrided and swabbed with povidone iodine (69b). The fish was also placed on systemic antibiotics (enrofloxacin, 10 mg/kg intraperitoneally every 48 hours for two weeks) to reduce the possibility of septicemia. The fish recovered uneventfully.

A practical alternative to MS-222 is clove oil. Clove oil is available over the counter at many pharmacies. Clove oil, also known as eugenol, is not completely soluble in water and should be diluted with ethanol at a rate of 1:10 (clove oil:ethanol) to yield a working stock solution of 100 mg/ml, since each ml of clove oil contains approximately 1 g of drug. Concentrations of between 40 and 120 mg/L are effective in freshwater and marine species and results are comparable to MS-222.

70 i. The photograph shows a symmetrical swelling of the abdomen with elevation of the scales to give a 'pine cone' appearance to the fish. There is also bilateral exophthalmos present.

The changes are those typical of 'dropsy' in which there is an upset in the fluid balance mechanisms with retention of fluid within the abdominal cavity and tissues. Tissue edema results in retrobulbar swelling which in turn produces the exophthalmos.

ii. Edema in other tissues may be apparent, as well as swelling of the vent or of bowel loops when examined at necropsy.

71 The ovary. The organization of the ovary varies in different species of teleosts (live-bearers versus egg-layers). The ovaries are paired or bilobed, elongate organs that are enclosed by a tunica albuginea containing smooth muscle and fibrous connective tissue and are suspended from the dorsal abdominal wall by the mesovaria.

72 An adult Queensland grouper (aged 25 years old and weighing about 180 kg) presents with trauma to its lower jaw and some abrasions over its left operculum. The animal has been eating well and its respiratory rate is within normal limits. Two other groupers in this exhibit appear normal. The aquarist reports that for the past several months the animal has been swimming around the tank predominantly to the left and will not accept food presented on its left side.

How could you evaluate this animal's visual capabilities?

73 An estuarine fish tank with a history of ectoparasite infestations is converted to a marine invertebrate tank, intended to house anemones and crabs. Within 24 hours of stocking the tank, all the animals die.

Propose a scenario to account for the rapid deaths, and explain how you would confirm your hypothesis.

74 Where is the anatomic location of the pancreas (**74**)?

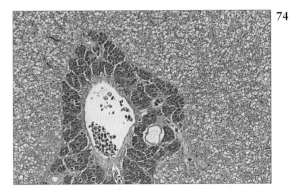
74

75 What is the ophthalmic condition shown in this mature koi (**75**)?

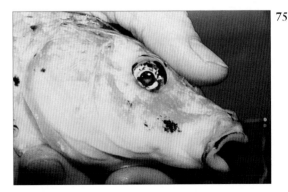
75

72a 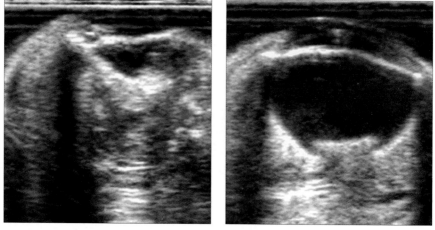 72b

72 Most fish react to even a dim light beam shown into their eyes. If no reaction is evident, a close physical examination is warranted. In this case a diver entered the animal's tank with a pressurized garden sprayer containing a solution of concentrated MS-222 (25 g/L). A small amount of dye such as methylene blue can be added to the solution to aid in visualizing the stream of anesthetic. The solution is then sprayed into the animal's mouth, which is 'inhaled' by the fish and passes over the gills. Induction usually occurs within five minutes. The cornea and lens of both eyes appeared normal and there were no other signs of abnormalities. Ultrasonographic examination is particularly useful in evaluating the fish patient provided that the scales are not too thick. In this case, ultrasonography revealed a large space-occupying mass in the posterior chamber of the left eye (**72a**). The right eye is apparently normal (**72b**). The etiology of this problem is unknown. The animal continues to be blind in the left eye but is otherwise normal.

73 The history of ectoparasites in the tank suggests the fish may have been treated with copper. Residual copper could attain concentrations lethal to invertebrates, particularly considering the conversion from low salinity estuary conditions to full marine salinity, because increased salinity releases adsorbed copper from the substrate. Determine the treatment history for the tank, and measure the free divalent copper ion concentration. Concentrations >0.01 p.p.m. are toxic for many invertebrates.

74 The location of the pancreas varies within and between species. The most common sites are within the mesenteric fat among the pyloric ceca or surrounding the portal vessels entering the liver (forming the hepatopancreas), or dispersed within the splenic capsule.

75 Lenticular cataract.

76 You are presented with a problem in which a high proportion of fish in a pond are collecting at the area below a waterfall and at the surface. What would be your provisional list of differentials, and how would you go about investigating the problem?

77 i. What is the probable nature of these lesions (77)?
ii. What is the prognosis?

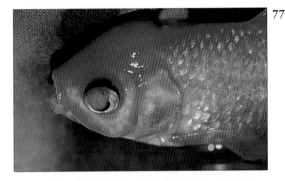

78 A new pet store owner calls and is concerned that his cory catfish (78) that he has just purchased from a wholesaler are sick because they are frequently swimming to the surface and then submerging. The fish are eating and none have died. What is the explanation?

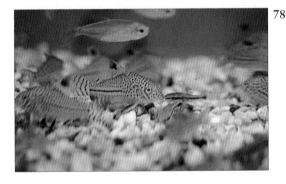

79 i. What vein is being used to obtain a blood sample from this carp (79)?
ii. What blood parasites can be found in this species?

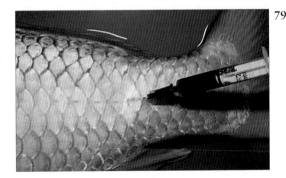

76 The fish are likely to be behaving in this way as there is a relatively higher concentration of dissolved oxygen in these areas. This behavior can be the result of any problem compromising the transport of oxygen to the tissues. This could include: low dissolved oxygen levels in the water caused by environmental factors (e.g. pollution, algal blooms, or high ambient temperatures with little shade); gill disease; anemia.

The possible environmental factors can be assessed by examination of the pond, measuring the water quality parameters (including dissolved oxygen), and a carefully taken history. Deoxygenation of the water can result from a large biological oxygen demand (BOD) which typically is caused by organic matter pollution. This debris requires a large quantity of oxygen when degraded by aerobic pathways. Overstocking with aquatic plants can produce reduced oxygen at night. Paradoxically, plants are used to improve the oxygen production by photosynthesis. This process requires light and ceases at night, whereas respiration continues. At this time there is a net requirement for oxygen causing a reduction in the amount available to the fish.

Algal blooms typically occur in ponds in the spring as the water temperature rises, aided by the relatively high levels of nutrients present as a result of the degradation of plant material through the winter. This may also cause a drop in dissolved oxygen at night, and some algae may directly damage the gill by toxin production or simply by physically clogging the gill surface.

Direct observation of the gills would indicate if there is any excessive mucus or signs of necrosis indicative of extensive bacterial or parasitic gill disease. Samples of the gill tips can be taken for microscopic examination from the live fish.

77 i. The photograph shows the gross appearance of a goldfish with raised nodules on the back of the neck and cornea. These are papillomas, small benign tumors of epithelial cell origin, which are common in many species of freshwater and marine fish.
ii. They are often multiple and have a predilection for the head region. They generally cause few clinical problems but are disfiguring. Surgical removal is an option.

78 This is normal behavior for most species belonging to this genus. They can gulp air and utilize it for respiration.

79 i. The caudal vein.
ii. *Sanguinicola inermis*, a digenean trematode; *Trypanosoma carassi*, a trypanosome; and *Trypanoplasma borreli*, a similar flagellate parasite.

80 This spiny puffer remained anorectic for 16 days (80). The fish was housed in a 600,000-L marine aquarium with numerous species of tropical marine fish. The water quality parameters were: temperature of 24°C (75.2°F), salinity of 32 p.p.t., pH 8.0, and dissolved oxygen of 6.0 p.p.m. The fish was removed from the main aquarium using a net and moved to an attached holding tank. The fish was anesthetized

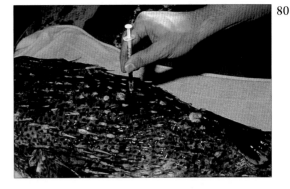

80

using 70 p.p.m. tricaine methanesulfonate (MS-222) and blood was collected for a blood profile. The fish was then tube fed 60 ml of fish gruel through a gastric tube. The blood profile appeared unremarkable. The treatment plan included tube feeding the fish under anesthesia twice a week for as long as it remained anorectic. After a week of treatment, the fish developed a swelling at the base of many of the spines. The swellings appeared to be associated with small abscesses and granulomas.
i. What is the most probable cause of the lesions at the base of the spines?
ii. How can this condition be prevented?
iii. What precaution should be made during anesthetic recovery of spiny puffers?

81 i. What are the organisms seen in the photograph (81)?
ii. With what clinical lesions are they associated?

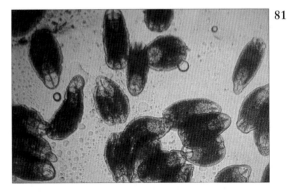

81

82 A pet store has set up a flow-through system using a large charcoal filter to pretreat incoming city water. Low-level mortalities have occurred regularly throughout the store, and despite assistance from fish health professionals, no infectious agents have been found. Finally, extensive water quality testing has been done and a residual chlorine level of 0.02 p.p.m. is detected.
i. Is this enough to cause the observed mortalities?
ii. What can be done immediately to stop these mortalities?

80 i. Using nets to capture spiny puffer fish results in damage to the spines as the fish inflates itself with water to extend its spines in self-defense. The fish becomes entangled in the net because of the extended spines. The netting material causes removal of the overlying skin resulting in exposure of the hard spine. The skin gathers at the base of the damaged spine in a manner similar to the rolling down of one's sock. This tissue becomes infected with opportunistic pathogenic micro-organisms.

ii. This condition can be prevented by avoiding the use of nets to catch this type of fish. A bucket can be used to capture the inflated fish without causing damage to the spines. In this case, the fish would begin to inflate as soon as it was approached by the aquarist. The aquarist would gently guide the poorly mobile inflated puffer into a large plastic trash container. Once captured, the fish was gently transferred to another plastic trash container containing 70 p.p.m. MS-222 for anesthesia. Anesthesia was required to relax the fish to allow passage of the stomach tube because the mouth is sealed closed in an inflated puffer fish. The fish was given amikacin (3.0 mg/kg intramuscularly every 72 hours) as treatment for the multiple cutaneous abscesses.

iii. During recovery from anesthesia, there is a risk that the puffer fish will inflate itself with air instead of water. Puffers inflate themselves by filling subcutaneous spaces with water. If they inflate with air, they will float to the surface and will be unable to submerge. It is difficult for the air-inflated puffer to remove the air and the fish may require assistance. If this should happen, the caudal end of the fish is pushed down into the water allowing the head to point upward. Air will escape through the mouth. This method of air removal is not always successful and the fish should be closely monitored. The exposed dorsal part of the fish should be kept wet until the fish expels the air on its own.

This fish responded to the antibiotic therapy and eventually began to eat on its own. The cause of the anorexia remained a mystery.

81 i. These organisms were found in the eye of a marine fish. They are metacercariae of the eye fluke (*Diplostomum* sp.).

ii. As its common name suggests, this organism has a predilection for the eye and may cause cataracts and blindness. The life cycle is completed when the secondary host in which the metacercariae are encysted is eaten by the specific primary host higher up the food chain.

82 i. Chlorine is highly toxic to fish. Concentrations of 0.02 p.p.m. can cause low-level mortality in a population, whereas concentrations of 0.04 p.p.m. can be 100% lethal. Municipal water supplies (out of the tap) usually contain between 1.0 and 2.0 p.p.m. chlorine. Residual chlorine can be easily identified using commercially available colormetric test kits.

ii. Sodium thiosulfate will remove chlorine immediately from aquatic systems. For each 1.0 p.p.m. chlorine present, 7.4 p.p.m. sodium thiosulfate should be added. Aeration must be maintained when sodium thiosulfate is introduced.

83 You have diagnosed a problem in some outdoor koi and need to medicate the pond. Unfortunately, the owner has no idea what the volume of the pond is. How can you calculate the volume of the pond without draining and refilling it?

84 The photograph shows a gross postmortem of a goldfish with the left abdominal wall removed (84). What lesions are visible?

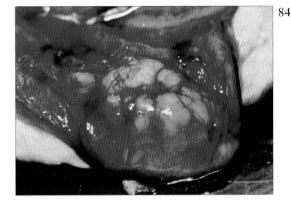
84

85 A slippery dick from a large marine exhibit aquarium is selected at random for routine health screening. A large bilateral nodular swelling at the base of the gills and extending upward along the lower gill arches is found. A histologic section is shown (85).
i. What is your diagnosis?
ii. What are some treatment options?

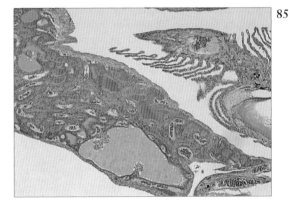
85

86 An aquarium owner has been using zeolite to counteract high ammonia levels in his newly purchased freshwater aquarium. He is changing water only sporadically. He reports that his fish continue to be sluggish and inappetent, and several have died in the last 24 hours, although his test kit shows an ammonia reading of zero. What characteristic of zeolite may be responsible for the problems in this aquarium?

83 The first method is to simply calculate the volume of the pond using the equation: volume = surface area × average depth. In order to calculate surface area, multiply the length by the width. For circular ponds, the equation for surface area is 3.14 × radius². For example, a rectangular pond 6 m long × 4 m wide would have a surface area of 24 sq m. A circular pond with a diameter (twice the radius) of 4 m would have a surface area of approximately 12.5 sq m. Calculating average depth can be difficult in a pond with a very uneven bottom. To keep things simple, assume that the average depth of both ponds is 1 m. Applying the above formula, the rectangular pond has a volume of 24 cu m and the circular pond 12.5 cu m. Since each cu m equals 1,000 liters, the rectangular pond contains 24,000 liters and the circular pond 12,500 liters.

This equation can also be applied to aquaria. You multiply length × depth × width to arrive at the volume. For example, an aquarium with inside measurements of 0.6 × 0.3 × 0.25 m would have a volume of 0.045 cu m. The aquarium contains 45 liters.

84 The photograph shows an ovoid mass in the ventral abdomen. The mass has distinct white nodules. There is also infiltration between the other abdominal viscera making it impossible to separate these structures. The mesentery is very hyperemic and inflamed, with distinct areas of hemorrhage.

The external appearance of the fish showed a swollen abdomen and hyperemia of the skin with elevated scales. These changes are consistent with a generalized septicemia/viremia/toxemia. *Aeromonas* was isolated from the kidney and was considered to be a secondary infection. The primary lesion was the abdominal mass, which histopathology proved to be an adenocarcinoma of the pancreatic tissue.

85 i. Thyroid hyperplasia (goiter). Eosinophilic colloid fills thyroid follicles of varying size and shape. Secondary lamellae of the gill are present at upper right. The thyroid of most fish is a diffuse organ located along the floor of the gill chamber, but thyroid tissue can also be found in the spleen, heart, and cranial kidney. Goiter may be difficult to distinguish from thyroid carcinoma, and was mistakenly described as such when initially found in salmonids on iodine-deficient diets.
ii. Iodine-deficiency goiter responds to iodine-replacement therapy. A primary iodine deficiency is unlikely in marine fish. Search for and eliminate goitrogenic substances in feed. A similar syndrome in sharks responds to thyroxine therapy, presumably by restoring the negative feedback loop on thyroid-releasing hormone and thyroid-stimulating hormone production.

86 Zeolite is not capable of removing nitrite from water. If frequent water changes are not performed during the break-in period, nitrite toxicity can develop in the face of negligible ammonia.

Note. Zeolite cannot remove ammonia from marine aquaria.

87 This leopard shark presented with a large ulcerative lesion near the tip of the tail (87). The shark was housed in a 150,000-L circular concrete aquarium with several other sharks, including blacktip reef sharks, whitetip reef sharks, nurse sharks, and juvenile brown sharks. A large guitarfish was also housed in the aquarium with the sharks. The typical behavior of this shark was to swim the perimeter of the aquarium close to the concrete walls.

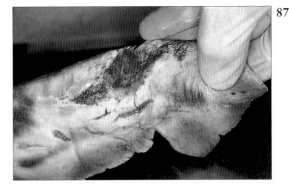

i. What are the possible causes for the cutaneous lesion?
ii. What course of treatment would you prescribe?

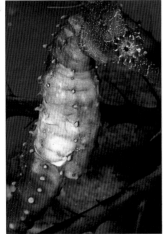

88 The pale areas on this seahorse are abnormal (88a). The lesion is caused by an external protozoal parasite.
i. What organisms are on your differential list?
ii. How would you confirm your diagnosis?

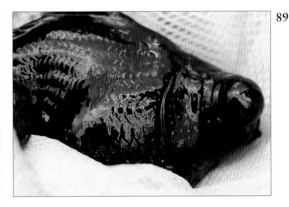

89 This mature black Moor goldfish presents because of pronounced, raised, 1-mm diameter nodules on the pectoral fins and opercula (89). The fish appears otherwise healthy and the owner has not experienced any losses in his aquarium. What is the explanation?

87 i. Traumatic injury should be high on the list of possible causes. This shark was housed with a number of potentially aggressive sharks and a bite is the most probable cause of the wound on the tail, based upon the appearance of the wound. Other possible etiologies would include bacterial, fungal, or parasitic disease; however, these are typically secondary disorders. A neoplasm would be a rare possibility.

ii. A complication in this case was the swimming pattern of the shark. Because this shark preferred to swim adjacent to the side of the circular pool, each movement of the tail resulted in contact between the wound and the concrete wall. It is nearly impossible to apply a protective bandage to the tail of a shark. Tape, adhesives, or other methods of fixing a bandage on the skin of a shark are usually irritating to the skin and result in further skin injury. Therefore, removal of the shark to another habitat (to remove the threat of aggressive sharks and to disrupt the swimming pattern of the shark) would be the first choice in the management of this case. Unfortunately, as is typical in such situations, no other aquarium was available. One method of keeping sharks away from the side of the pool is to suspend plastic pipes that nearly reach the bottom of the pool in a vertical fashion at intervals that will disrupt the sharks' swimming pattern. Use of less abrasive material on the pool walls would also minimize damage to the skin. A broad-spectrum antibiotic should be considered in the treatment of deep wounds in sharks as a precaution against the development of bacteremia or septicemia. Antibiotics such as amikacin (2.5–3.0 mg/kg intramuscularly every 72 hours), enrofloxacin (5 mg/kg orally every 4 hours), or chloramphenicol (25–50 mg/kg orally once daily) have been used in sharks.

88 i. *Brooklynella hostilis*; *Uronema marinum.*

ii. Wet mounts of skin and fin biopsies should be examined immediately since many protozoal organisms die quickly and lose their characteristic morphology. This seahorse had a severe *Brooklynella* infestation. Living parasites are ciliated, heart-shaped and measure approximately 50 microns in diameter. This parasite has been dried and stained (**88b**). *Brooklynella* affects many species of marine fish, especially clownfish.

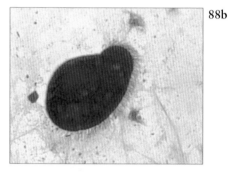

88b

Infections occur in crowded conditions and/or in debilitated fish. Prevention of the disease is directed at identification and treatment during quarantine. Short baths in freshwater (five minutes) will kill the parasites. Combinations of formaldehyde and malachite green have been used for aquarium treatments at a final concentration of 15–25 p.p.m. formalin and 0.05 p.p.m. malachite green.

89 During the spring breeding season, male goldfish develop nuptial tubercles on the surfaces of the opercula and pectoral fins. Grossly, these nodules can resemble the encysted stage of *Ichthyophthirius multifiliis*. This condition is normal.

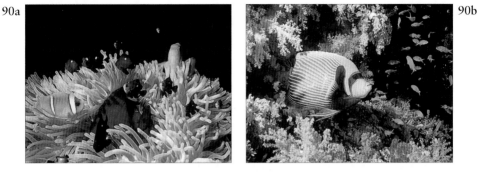

90 An owner has a 200-L aquarium that has held a stable population of marine aquarium fish for the past several months (90a, b). This includes four 5-cm blue damselfish, six 5-cm percula clownfish, and a 12-cm Emperor angelfish. There was no history of any morbidity or mortality in the aquarium during this time. One week ago, the owner introduced a 5-cm French angelfish into the aquarium. Today, the owner found the newly introduced angelfish in the corner of the aquarium and nearly dead. All the other fish appeared clinically normal. Upon presentation to the clinician, water quality examination revealed a temperature of 26°C (78.8°F) (obtained from history), total ammonia nitrate of 0 p.p.m, nitrite of <0.1 p.p.m., and pH of 8.1. Physical examination of the moribund angelfish showed frayed fins and several foci of depigmentation on the flanks. No pathogens were visible in wet mounts of skin or gills. Necropsy results were within normal limits. No bacteria were recovered from kidney culture.
i. What is the most probable cause of this problem?
ii. How would you treat this condition?

91 This pearl cichlid presented for multiple erosions of the head, which can be seen ventral to the eye and dorsal to the mouth (91).
i. What is this condition called?
ii. What are some probable causes of this syndrome?
iii. How would you manage this problem?

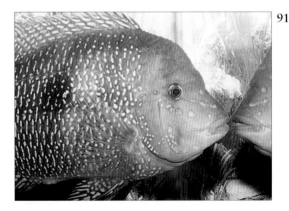

92 Does infection of fish with mycobacteria pose a threat to human health?

90 i. The absence of any pathogens in the skin wounds and lack of any discernible infectious agent upon necropsy strongly indicates that the fish was the target of aggression by its tankmates. The owner should be queried thoroughly to see if there was any evidence of this event. The larger angelfish was probably the most significant source of this aggression, but the other fish may have also contributed to attacks.

ii. An attacked fish should be immediately placed into a separate quarantine tank to allow it to recover from its wounds. Prophylactic antibiotics may be used to prevent secondary bacterial infections if lesions are very deep or extensive. Most marine reef fish are highly territorial. This territoriality is usually displayed most aggressively against members of their same species. For solitary species such as angelfish, it is best not to have more than one individual of the same species in the tank. It is often inadvisable to even have more than one individual of the same Family. Fish that naturally school together, such as damselfish, can be kept as a group, but it is important to have at least three to four members of this group to avoid one dominant individual from constantly harassing only one other member of the group. When introducing any new individual into a tank with a well-established dominance hierarchy, it is best to gradually acclimate the fish to the population. This can be done by placing the newly introduced fish into a clear container that is suspended into the tank. Keep the fish in this container for at least several days before releasing it into the aquarium.

91 i. Freshwater 'hole in the head' disease or head and lateral line erosion (HLLE). The syndrome does differ between freshwater and marine species.

ii. These lesions have been linked to poor water quality, inadequate nutrition, protozoal ectoparasites (*Hexamita* or *Spironucleus*), and a variety of bacterial pathogens.

iii. Proper management would include a thorough evaluation of the water quality parameters as well as lesion scrapings and culture. Treatment would progress according to diagnostic findings. This fish had a history of improving slightly after metronidazole was administered to the water (6 p.p.m.) by the owners. The fish lived for several years with the lesions and was finally killed painlessly when it became debilitated and stopped eating at the age of nine years. Necropsy findings included systemic mycobacteriosis and mycobacterial involvement of the erosive lesions.

92 The two most common species of mycobacteria affecting fish are *Mycobacterium marinum* and *Mycobacterium fortuitum*. The former has been associated with hypersensitivity reactions of the skin of humans. Because the bacterium does not grow at 37°C (98.6°F), systemic spread does not occur. *Mycobacterium fortuitum* tolerates a wider temperature range, and local abscesses caused by this organism have been described in humans.

93 A pet store owner has lost 30% of his marine fish in the past five days and the surviving fish are extremely lethargic. Some have been seen 'coughing' (backflushing water across the gills) and rubbing the operculum along objects in the tank. Some have a shimmering golden appearance along the dorsal body surface. None are eating very well. All the marine fish are housed in a 5,700-L re-circulating system. There is no

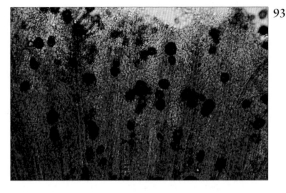

ozonation or ultraviolet sterilization of system water. A moribund percula clownfish is submitted for examination. Gill biopsy reveals massive numbers of *Amyloodinium* on the lamellae (93). Moderate numbers are present on skin scrapings.

i. What can the pet retailer do to salvage the fish that are sick?
ii. Given two treatment options (copper and chloroquine), discuss the advantages and disadvantages of each.
iii. Is there anything that can be done to prevent this problem in the future?

94 Known as 'feather dusters,' these invertebrates will occasionally shed their 'feathers,' which can regrow (94). What are these feathers, and why are they shed?

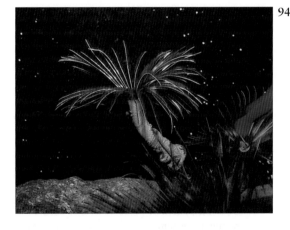

95 Discuss methods of euthanasia recommended to professional fisheries personnel as well as home hobbyists.

93 i. Given the situation presented – 30% mortality rate over a 5-day period, and examined fish heavily infested with *Amyloodinium* – salvaging the fish remaining in the store may be difficult. In the author's experience, the treatment of choice would be chloroquine at 10.0 p.p.m. The chemical can be added to the entire 5,700-L system and fish should begin to improve almost immediately. The other option would be to add 0.2 p.p.m. copper ion (Cu^{2+}) to the system for three weeks. Any invertebrates would need to be removed from the system before copper addition.

ii. The main disadvantage of chloroquine treatment is that it is not approved for use in any aquatic species in the USA. The compound is an antimalarial, and, under experimental conditions, has provided excellent control of *Amyloodinium* in red drum. Copper has been used as a parasiticide in marine systems for many years. An important disadvantage to using copper in the situation described is that the fish are severely compromised (i.e. fish which are very sick and heavily infected with *Amyloodinium* do not tolerate copper well). In addition, maintaining active copper (Cu^{2+}) concentrations of 0.2 p.p.m. can be labor intensive. Copper concentration should be checked several times a day and additional copper may need to be added to the system.

iii. The occasional introduction of undesirable infectious agents into a pet store is not completely preventable. At the very least, incoming fish should be dipped in freshwater (marine fish) or sea water (freshwater fish). Additionally, a system such as the one described should have some means of sanitizing water before it recirculates back to the tanks. A properly installed and maintained ultraviolet light unit can do a reasonable job of preventing the transmission of infectious agents from one tank to another.

94 Feather dusters are polychaete worms belonging to a group known as the fan worms (Sabellidae). The fan, or feathers, are termed radioles; they are used both for filter feeding and gaseous exchange, and they encircle the mouth. Trapped food particles are passed down towards the mouth by ciliary action. Each radiole has a single blood vessel with a regular alternating blood flow. The worm itself produces a parchment-like tube in which it resides. The radioles are shed usually as a response to poor water quality, or some other stressor.

95 Veterinarians often must recommend to a client that a fish be euthanatized. Several methods of fish euthanasia are approved by the American Veterinary Medical Association (AVMA) including: cranial concussion followed by decapitation; cervical dislocation followed by double pithing (both the brain and spinal cord); chemical overdose. If available, tricaine methanesulfonate (TMS) at a dose of 300–500 p.p.m. for 15 minutes will kill most fish. Since most hobbyists and veterinary clinics do not have TMS on hand, alternatives include benzocaine hydrochloride, oil of cloves, and even carbon dioxide in the form of antacid tablets (2–3 tablets/L of water). Injectable sodium pentobarbital (60 mg/kg) given IV or IP is another chemical alternative for larger fish. As a last resort, a client in a remote location can use ethanol at a final concentration of 10%. Veterinarians should consider offering a euthanasia service since many clients are attached to their fish pets.

96 Describe how you would carry out a routine postmortem examination when investigating disease in a fish.

97 This Midas cichlid is in the process of eating a sinking food pellet (97). An enlarged area is present in the dorsal cranial area of this fish. What is its cause?

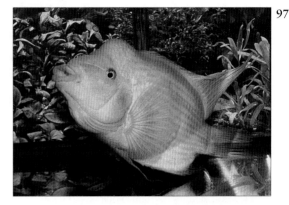

97

98 This figure is a transverse section CT scan of a normal koi just caudal to the eyes (98). Identify the labeled structures.

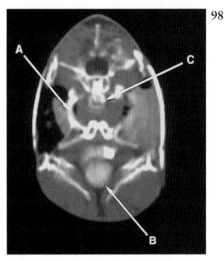

98

99 Which of the following is *not* a consequence of positioning an aquarium in direct sunlight?
A Increased rate of algae growth.
B Increased rate of fish growth.
C Increased fish stress.
D Daily temperature fluctuations.

96 The clinical examination of live fish is limited by their aquatic environment and by the relatively narrow range and non-specificity of clinical signs. Post-mortem and laboratory investigations are therefore essential in the diagnosis of fish disease and it is often necessary to sacrifice an affected individual in a population to carry out these investigations.

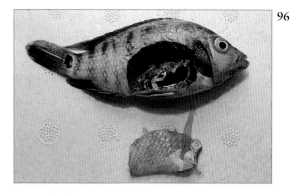

After obtaining a detailed clinical history, affected individuals should be examined for external abnormalities – scale loss and ulcers, hemorrhage, fin and tail erosion, eye abnormalities, gill damage, abdominal swellings, grossly visible parasites or fungal infection (changes in pigmentation and over-production of mucus are often more noticeable while the fish is in the water). Skin scrapes and gill biopsies should be examined for the presence of parasites and other disease processes.

The abdomen of the fish should be opened along the ventral midline, taking care not to puncture the gastrointestinal tract (96). The presence of abdominal fluid, hemorrhage, or both, should be noted.

The abdominal organs should be examined for abnormalities and the presence of grossly visible parasites.

At this point the kidney can be exposed aseptically and a sample of kidney tissue obtained for bacteriologic examination.

Tissue samples can be taken for histopathologic examination and the gut and stomach opened and examined for the presence of parasites.

If a toxic insult or viral infection is suspected, contact a specialized laboratory to discuss the most appropriate diagnostic procedures.

97 This is a normal condition. Midas cichlids are New World cichlids. Most species belonging to this group are sexually dimorphic; mature males have a pronounced hump or mass on their head.

98 The labeled structures are as follows:
A. Gill arch.
B. Cardiac ventricle.
C. Pharyngeal tooth.

99 B. Because of the stress caused by fluctuations in temperature, fish growth may actually be retarded. Temperature fluctuations may cause immunosuppression, rendering fish susceptible to infections and further hindering growth.

100 A hobbyist has purchased two *Leporinus* fish from a local pet supplier. On close inspection in her home aquarium, she observes small white spots primarily on the dorsal fin of the fish (**100**). A few of the white spots are located on the tail fin, and a few are located on the body. The fish are active, eating, and appear to be otherwise normal. The owner

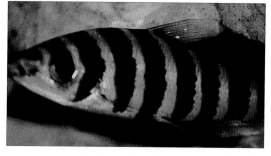

has had the fish for two weeks in her mixed community aquarium. You have seen the fish and verify that the spots are present and vary in size from 1–2 mm in diameter. The cysts appear to be deeply embedded in the skin.

i. What disease entities should be considered when white spots are identified on a fish?

ii. Which of the above differentials can be tentatively ruled out based on the clinical presentation and history?

iii. How can the tentative diagnosis be confirmed?

iv. Is the condition infectious to other fish in the aquarium?

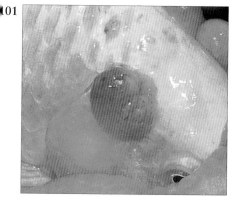

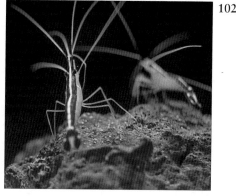

101 This fish was presented with a large sessile mass on its head that had been present for three years (**101**).

i. What type of lesion is this likely to be?

ii. What course of action is required?

102 How are these candy-striped shrimp beneficial to fish in a marine aquarium (**102**)?

103 How should commercial fish foods be stored?

100 i. (1) Sporozoan cysts; (2) colonies of the dinoflagellate *Oodinium* (velvet disease); encysted metacercaria; (3) colonies of *Epistylis*; (4) mucus tabs resulting from external parasites; (5) mature stages of *Ichthyophthirius multifiliis*.
ii. You have thought about most of the common disease entities which could affect a fish. You exclude *Ichthyophthirius* because the cysts on the fish have remained in the same location and the other fish have not become infected. Oodiniasis is also excluded for the same reasons; additionally, fish affected with *Oodinium* will have a white to yellow dusty appearance rather than discrete spots. Metacercaria are encysted forms of digenetic trematodes where aquatic birds are the final host. You have excluded these by the fact that cysts are usually large (2–3 mm) and protrude from the surface of the skin. *Epistylis* is a possibility, but colonies of the epiphytic stalked protozoans appear as large tufts (3–4 mm) growing from the surface of the skin rather than circumscribed cysts. Small white spots as described could be cysts of one of the many species of sporozoan parasites which affect fish. Embedded cysts on the surface of a fish, which do not affect the behavior of the fish and are not observed to be infectious to other fish in the aquarium, should suggest the presence of a sporozoan disease.
iii. The fish should be captured, restrained and/or anesthetized, and a scraping made of the area of the cyst. In this case, a diagnosis of the sporozoan *Henneguya* sp. was confirmed. An examination of wet mounts using a ×40 objective would reveal hundreds of elongated spores with two tail extensions. *Henneguya* infections are quite common in striped *Leporinus*.
iv. The life cycle of this parasite is unknown. Based on other well-known cycles, an intermediate host such as an oligochaete may be required for transmission. Clinical experience suggests that other fish will not be infected. Affected fish usually remain clinically healthy.

101 i. A papilloma.
ii. These are common neoplasms and often do not require treatment. Many will periodically slough and leave a relatively normal but hyperplastic surface; however, the tumors may then spontaneously recur. Such events suggest that a virus may be involved, and other parts of the fish may also be affected. If these tumors affect vital areas such as the mouth or opercula, surgical removal is indicated. Total excision is rarely possible and regrowth of the tumor may occur.

102 Like many reef shrimp, they are 'cleaners', and can actually remove parasites and cellular debris from certain species of fish.

103 Commercial flake and pelleted foods should be stored in tightly sealed containers in either the refrigerator or freezer (the cooler the temperature the better). Warmer storage temperatures lead to oxidation and the formation of free radicals. When this happens, vitamins such as A and C are destroyed. At higher temperatures, sugars and amino acids may form complexes, rendering important proteins inactive. Hobbyists should be encouraged to purchase small containers of food, no larger than can be consumed by the fish in a six-month period.

104 As the veterinarian in the region most known for treating pet fish, you are hired as a consultant by the planning committee for a new public aquarium to be built in your city. It is a highly political project, and everyone hopes it will revitalize the decaying downtown area. The director of a major established aquarium is also a consultant and the large freshwater and saltwater displays being planned will be spectacular, but when you review the plans you do not see any hospital or quarantine space, or tanks for reservoir water (for water changes). All of the displays are connected together on a single recirculating system.
i. What would be your recommendations for a reasonable amount of reservoir water to maintain?
ii. What quarantine should be implemented in the aquarium and how much space will be required?

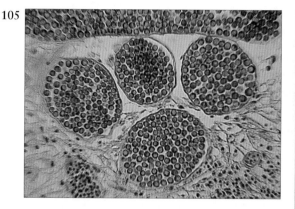

105

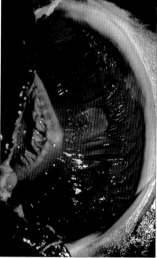

106

105 Histologic examination of an 8-mm skin lump removed from a koi revealed many of these cystic structures full of spherical objects in the dermis (PAS staining, ×400) (**105**).
What is the cause of the lesion?

106 Describe the disease condition illustrated by the photograph (**106**).

104 i. When water must be processed before use, it is critical to have reservoirs containing conditioned water for routine and emergency water changes. If exhibits will hold water of varying salinities and temperatures, it may be appropriate to have multiple reservoirs; otherwise, delays in water replacement can be catastrophic. The minimum reservoir volume should hold 50% of the volume of water that will be holding fish. This allows for the worst case scenario of a need to make a 50% water change on all systems at once. This might occur with a severe contamination problem. Rarely is there funding to provide for this much reservoir space, but, as a consultant, you should stand by the need for optimal reservoir size.

ii. It is surprisingly easy for the excitement over new exhibits and displays to cause even experienced planners to forget that aquatic animals can become ill. The long incubation period of several fish diseases makes relatively long quarantines appropriate to protect very valuable display collections. A routine minimum quarantine is six weeks, but even this may be too short and planners may not realize that in an all-in, all-out quarantine, disease outbreaks will extend routine six-week quarantines to several months. Adequate space to hold fish outside the exhibit for these periods must be designed into the building. The amount of space will depend very much on the number of displays and the number of species being exhibited. Plans to conduct initial quarantines in other facilities to speed the opening of the aquarium should not be allowed to supplant the construction of quarantine facilities to continually supplement the exhibits. Quarantine facilities for very large species are rarely constructed because of their cost. Everyone should be aware that this compromise almost always results in major problems later in the operation of the facility.

Although routine mortality should not exceed 10% of the collection per year, wise curators will want to hold the fish (already quarantined) required to replace at least two or three of the exhibits should a sudden catastrophe strike. Quarantine facilities should be sufficient to allow full quarantine of all replacement stock without using back-holding space dedicated for supporting healthy fish ready to go on exhibit.

105 Infection with *Dermocystidium koi*. The large cystic structures are cross-section views through the fungal hyphae which are packed with spores. The latter contain a large central vacuole or refractile body with the cytoplasm and nucleus restricted to the narrow periphery. This gives the spores a characteristic 'signet-ring' appearance.

106 The photograph shows a discrete, oval, raised, plaque-like lesion on the gill of a koi carp recently imported to the UK from Japan. These changes were consistent with a diagnosis of branchiomycosis (gill rot), which is a disease of freshwater fish caused by the fungus *Branchiomyces*. It has been described in Europe, Japan, India, and parts of the USA. Spores attach to the gill surface and germinate to form hyphae. These hyphae proliferate, causing damage to the blood supply and necrosis. Sloughing of this necrotic tissue releases spores into the water, which then continue to develop on the floor of the pond or aquarium if conditions are favorable (i.e. temperatures of 25–32°C (77.0–89.6°F), high levels of organic material, low oxygen levels, and a low pH).

107 With regard to the disease in 106:
i. What tests can be performed to confirm the diagnosis?
ii. How is the organism transmitted, and what measures would you advise to treat and prevent the problem?

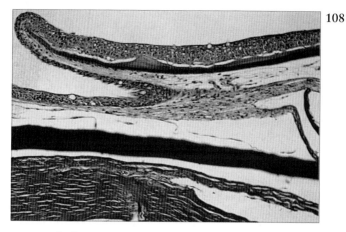

108 What structure is shown (108)? Is it normal to see small numbers of leukocytes within this structure?

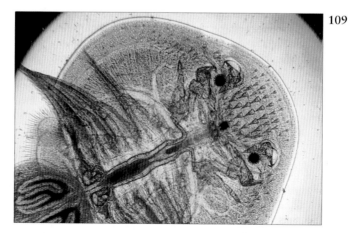

109 i. What is the common name of this parasite (×20) (109)?
ii. What is its genus?
iii. How does it feed?
iv. What are the major clinical concerns with this parasite?

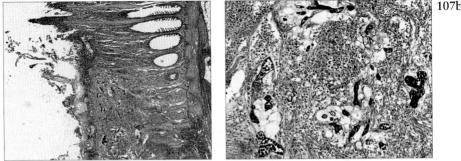

107a

107b

107 i. The diagnosis of branchiomycosis could be confirmed by examining fresh scrapings taken from the lesion and by histopathology. In this particular case, the scraping would be expected to yield branched aseptate hyphae. Large areas of necrosis containing fungal spores and hyphae can be seen on histopathology with a GMS (Gomori methenamine silver) preparation (**107a, b**).
ii. Fungal spores can be introduced directly by adding infected or carrier fish, or indirectly by birds or the use of raw fish products.

Treatment is generally unrewarding, although 2-phenoxyethanol has been suggested. Control is achieved by good hygiene, avoiding the use of raw fish products, and adequate quarantine of all new fish to avoid introduction of the organism.

108 This fish skin is composed of an epidermis, a dermis, and in some areas, a hypodermis. The scale (bright eosinophilic hyaline structure) lies in a scale pocket that is overlaid by dermis (stratum compactum). There may be small numbers of leukocytes within the stratum spongiosum of the dermis. In addition to epithelial cells, there are also mucus cells that secrete the important protective mucus covering. Melanophores are usually found within the dermis or in the hypodermis and less commonly in the epidermis. Some fish (e.g. catfish) also have large prominent polyhedral cells in the epidermis that have large to moderate amounts of eosinophilic cytoplasm and a centrally placed nucleus. These are alarm cells (or Schrekstoffzellen), which secrete an alarm or 'fright' substance when the epidermis is damaged.

109 i. The fish louse.
ii. *Argulus.*
iii. This parasite feeds by piercing the skin with its sharp stylet (visible along the ventral midline of the animal) and then sucking up body fluids with its mouth parts.
iv. Although a light *Argulus* infection is rarely fatal, the parasites irritate the skin, making the fish stressed and uncomfortable. A heavy fish louse infestation may allow opportunistic pathogens to infect the host, and fish lice are known directly to transmit bacterial and viral diseases.

110 Which of the following anesthetic agents should you choose for an exploratory coeliotomy in a red oscar?

- Carbon dioxide.
- Halothane.
- Ketamine hydrochloride.
- Quinaldine sulfate.
- Tricaine methanesulfonate (MS-222).

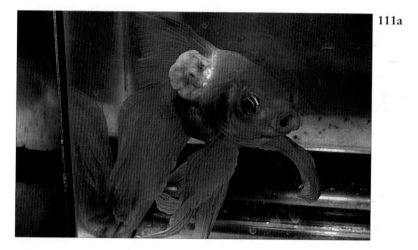

111a

111 This goldfish has a history of a slowly developing polypoid soft-tissue mass on the dorsum that sometimes is abraded and bleeds (**111a**). What is your diagnosis, and how would you treat this condition?

112 When is anesthesia or sedation indicated in the piscine patient?

110 Although each of the compounds listed has been used as an anesthetic in fish, the best choice among these for the procedure specified is tricaine methanesulfonate. Carbon dioxide can be used to achieve anesthesia in fish. As with halothane, the amount delivered to the fish can be difficult to control. Carbon dioxide also affords little or no muscle relaxation, which is desirable when performing a coeliotomy. Halothane is an effective anesthetic agent in mammals; however, it is difficult to control the concentration delivered to fish. Also, human exposure to halothane gas that escapes from the water can cause concern. Ketamine has been used effectively as a fish anesthetic; however, it is difficult to maintain a surgical anesthetic plane for prolonged periods with injectable anesthetic agents. Quinaldine sulfate can be administered in a very controlled fashion to the piscine patient. Quinaldine is superior to tricaine in that it is less expensive and has a wider margin of safety. Unfortunately, quinaldine sulfate does not suppress reflex motion and fish anesthetized with this compound often move in response to touch.

111 Based on the history and gross appearance, the most likely diagnosis is a neoplastic mass (with granulomas and benign hyperplasia on the differential list). In this case, the tumor is a fibrosarcoma (111b). In some fish, neoplasia has a viral etiology and may occur seasonally (i.e. appear and then regress spontaneously). There are several reports of sarcomas in goldfish but no etiology has been con-firmed. If the mass does not impede the fish's movement, one could leave the mass or resect it (after confirming the diagnosis by biopsy). Wide excision may be necessary to prevent recurrence.

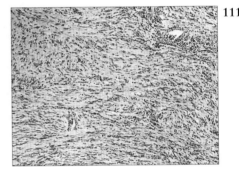

111b

112 Sedation or anesthesia might not be indicated when the procedures to be per-formed are minimally stressful (e.g. skin, gill, and fin biopsies of small patients) and can be done with physical restraint alone. Also, sedation or anesthesia might be con-traindicated in the severely debilitated patient. Sedation is indicated when the patient is easily stressed by handling and when minimal movement is desired (e.g. radiographing a large koi (112)). Anes-thesia is indicated for all procedures that require long periods without movement, invasive procedures (e.g. coeliotomy), any painful procedure, and in any fish that is refractory to sedation.

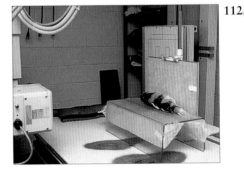

112

113 A hobbyist has treated her clown loaches prophylactically for *Ichthyophthirius multifiliis* with 0.1 p.p.m. malachite green. She repeated the treatment two days later and now fish are dying. Water quality parameters are within normal limits. A photomicrograph of a gill biopsy of an affected fish is shown (**113**).
i. What is the most probable explanation for the death of the clown loaches?
ii. What should be done?

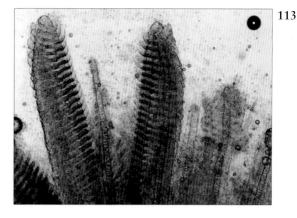

114 A 75-L aquarium contains nine neon tetras, two pearl gouramis, two cory catfish, and a *Plecostomus*. The owner reports that all the fish were purchased six days ago and placed in a newly acquired aquarium with fresh dechlorinated water and fresh filter material. In the past 24 hours, four of the tetras have died and several others have whitened fin edges.

Filtration consists of an outside power filter with disposable carbon-filled filter packs. No water changes have been performed to date.

Water quality parameters are as follows:

Temperature = 26°C (68°F)
pH = 7.4
Ammonia = 3.0 p.p.m.
Nitrite = 2.0 p.p.m.
Nitrate = 2.5 p.p.m.
Hardness = 130 p.p.m.

i. Based on the history and water quality information, what is the most likely diagnosis?
ii. What treatments are indicated?

115 i. Describe the lesion (**115**).
ii. What is the most probable disease organism involved?
iii. Are other factors likely to be implicated in the disease?

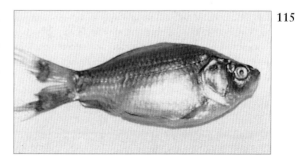

113 i. Scaleless fish, including clown loaches and catfish, are extremely sensitive to malachite green toxicity. The second treatment compounded damage done by the first chemical application, and significant destruction of secondary gill lamellae has resulted (113). Mortalities are probably secondary to inappropriate chemical treatment.

ii. Surviving fish should be maintained in clean water and not exposed to further chemical stress. Clown loaches are best treated for *I. multifiliis* by temperature manipulation. In the example given, there is no evidence that fish actually had an *I. multifiliis* problem. The owner should be educated on proper chemical use and quarantine protocols.

114 i. The likely diagnosis is 'new tank syndrome.' When a large number of fish are added to a system with no established bacterial flora, the nitrifying capacity of the system can be quickly overwhelmed, causing increases in the concentrations of toxic nitrogenous compounds. This may result in sluggish or inappetent fish, greatly increased susceptibility to infection, or sudden death. This situation can be averted by 'priming' the system with gravel or filter media from an established aquarium, introducing a very small number of fish until the biofilter is established, and daily monitoring of water parameters with water changes as needed to maintain acceptable levels of nitrogenous compounds, especially ammonia and nitrite.

ii. Immediate treatment may consist of:

- Daily 50% water changes until the un-ionized ammonia concentration is below 0.1 p.p.m.
- Addition of conditioned gravel or filter media to increase the rate at which colonization of the biofilter takes place.
- Addition of sodium chloride at 100 p.p.m. to decrease osmotic stress and decrease nitrite uptake by the fish.
- Addition of ammonia absorbing compounds to the filter.
- Specific treatment of opportunistic infections as indicated.

115 i. The photograph shows the gross appearance of the typical 'fin rot' lesion. This is part of a syndrome referred to as 'cold-water disease' as it is seen most commonly at temperatures of 4–10°C (39–50°F). The lesion shows erosion and loss of the distal section of the fin with swelling and necrosis at the advancing edge of the infection. As the disease organism spreads, the base of the tail (caudal peduncle) may become affected.

ii. The most commonly isolated organism is *Cytophaga psychrophila*, although other flexibacteria as well as *Aeromonas* and *Pseudomonas* are sometimes involved.

iii. Generally, this condition represents an opportunistic infection that is secondary to poor environmental conditions, nutritional problems, or physical damage. Once the infection is established it will spread to healthy tissue on the same fish and will become a source of infection to other fish in the pond.

Treatment is aimed at correcting the underlying stress factors. Parenteral antibiotics are of little value, although surface-active agents such as acriflavine and benzalkonium chloride added to the water may help. Raising the water temperature may help because *Cytophaga psychrophila* does not grow at temperatures above 12°C (53.6°F).

116 An established 200-L aquarium contains one 15-cm oscar, two 12-cm Jack Dempseys, a 12-cm *Plecostomus*, and an 18-cm albino channel catfish. Filtration consists of an external power filter with a carbon insert and an undergravel filter with two powerheads. Water is changed sporadically.

The owner complains that the fish are inappetent and lethargic with clamped fins, and that the water has a yellow–brown tinge and strange odor. Water quality parameters are as follows:

Temperature = 24°C (75.2°F)
Ammonia = 0.75 p.p.m.
Nitrite = 2.0 p.p.m.
pH = 5.8

A large amount of sediment has accumulated in the gravel overlying the under-gravel filter.

What is the likely diagnosis?

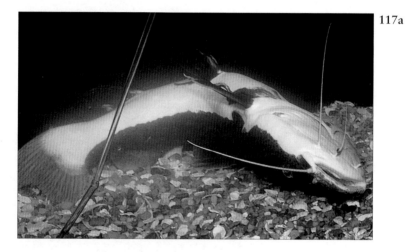
117a

117 A four-year-old redtail catfish kept in a 530-L tank began to develop mild fin necrosis about six weeks ago. The owner has treated the fish with antibiotics, first with a two-week course of tetracycline added to the water at 400 p.p.m. and then a kanamy-cin water treatment for the entire tank at 100 p.p.m. A day after the kanamycin treatment, the redtail catfish was found on its back with a swollen abdomen (**117a**). You conduct water analysis of the tank and find total ammonia to be 1.0 p.p.m. and nitrite to exceed the limits of your test kit, which is 4.0 p.p.m.
i. What is your diagnosis?
ii. What would be your treatment plan?

116 Improper cleaning of gravel during water changes and the subsequent accumulation of waste material increases the concentration of organic molecules responsible for discoloration and odor. The accumulation of sediment may also create areas of uneven water flow and decreased oxygenation in the undergravel filter bed, decreasing filter efficiency and predisposing to the formation of toxic nitrogen and sulfur compounds from anaerobic pockets in the bed. Abrupt changes in pH may also occur because of the accumulation of organic compounds.

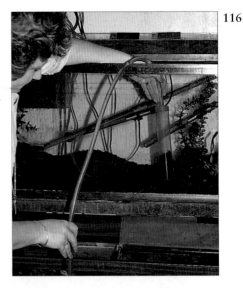

Prevention of recurrence should involve regular cleaning of the gravel substrate with a distended-end siphon tube (116) during water changes, and regular changes of filter carbon (if present), which can trap organic molecules and keep water clear and odor-free.

Note. Some experienced hobbyists recommend against the use of undergravel filters when keeping large cichlids or ornamental goldfish. Their messy eating habits and propensity to rearrange gravel may make maintenance of an undergravel filter difficult.

117 i. Nitrite toxicity, probably secondary to destruction of the biological filter with the administrations of antibiotics directly in the tank water.

ii. Immediate institution of daily 50% water changes is warranted in this case. Adding sodium chloride to achieve 100 p.p.m. will reduce uptake of nitrite. A 23-gauge butterfly catheter was used to remove 160 cm^3 of air from the swim

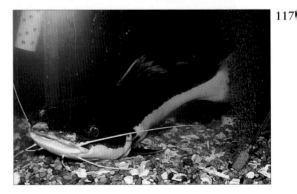

bladder and the fish was able to right itself (117b). It is not known what caused this swim bladder condition.

118 Several discus housed in a display aquarium have recently demonstrated depressed appetite, weight loss, and general darkening (**118**). The aquarium has a volume of 209 L, with an undergravel filter, and has been set up for about eight months. There are three medium-sized, powder blue discus in the display, as well as a plecostomous catfish for algae control. Water quality parameters are listed below:

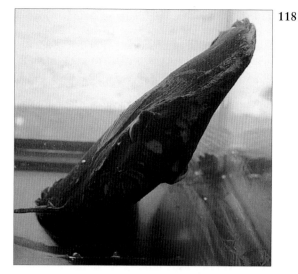
118

Dissolved oxygen: 7.4 p.p.m.
Total ammonia: 0.5 p.p.m.
Temperature: 30°C (86°F)
pH: 7.2
Total alkalinity: 60 p.p.m.
Nitrite: 0 p.p.m.
Total hardness: 50 p.p.m.

Gill and skin biopsies were negative and a large number of motile protozoans were visible in fecal smears.
i. What is the most probable cause of the depression and weight loss observed in the discus?
ii. What is the treatment of choice?
iii. What management practices should be put in place to prevent future problems?

119 A six-year-old cichlid requires surgery to repair an apparent deformity of its swim bladder. The surgeon estimates the time of surgery to be two hours. Tricaine methanesulfonate is the only anesthetic agent available.
i. How will you deliver the anesthetic to the fish during surgery?
ii. The surgeon complains that there is water flowing across the surgical field, along the ventral abdomen. How can you modify your procedure to eliminate this problem without reducing your flow rate?

118 i. *Spironucleus* (*Hexamita*) is a diplomonad flagellate that lives in the intestinal tract of many species of fish. Discus and angelfish are particularly susceptible to *Spironucleus*-related problems. Although diagnosis is possible from a fecal smear, a negative smear does not necessarily mean that the flagellates are not present. Wet mounts of intestinal contents are more useful for diagnostic purposes but sacrifice of the affected fish is required.

ii. Metronidazole is the treatment of choice for *Spironucleus* problems in ornamental fish. If fish are eating, metronidazole can be fed at a rate of 50 mg/kg (approximately 2.0 g active drug per kg of food). If fish are anoretic, metronidazole baths have demonstrated efficacy in angelfish. A concentration of 6 p.p.m. (approximately 250 mg in 38 L of water) administered every other day for three treatments is effective. Water changes should be performed between treatments. Often fish will begin eating after the first bath treatment. They can then be fed the medicated feed, which is less expensive and less labor intensive because the need for water changes is eliminated.

iii. Prophylactic treatment with metronidazole every three to six months is a sound management practice for many cichlids, particularly breeding stock. Discus in particular are extremely sensitive to changes in water quality and temperature. In the situation described above, there is no indication of which factors may have contributed to the *Spironucleus* outbreak; however, occasional treatment (every three to six months) with a metronidazole-medicated feed should be a routine practice for discus owners.

119 i. Because of the length of the procedure, continuous delivery of the anesthetic agent is required. This can be achieved in the following two ways. A large syringe may be used to manually force water through the mouth and over the gills of the fish. Using this method, water leaving the fish should trickle down into a pan to be readministered; otherwise, a

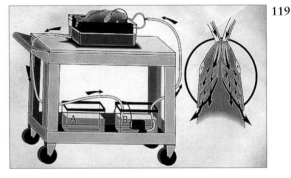

119

sufficient volume of anesthetic-containing water should be available for the surgery and the collecting pan should be periodically drained. Alternatively, an automated system can be assembled in which a small pump delivers anesthetic-containing water, via tubes, through the fish's mouth and over its gills (**119**). The water then trickles into a catch pan and flows back to a reservoir to be readministered to the fish. Flow rates may be adjusted by use of in-line valves. Drug concentrations may be changed by the addition of water or anesthetic to the reservoir.

ii. To solve the problem of water flowing over the surgical field without reducing the flow rate, the anesthetic-containing water can be delivered from the opercular cavity into the buccal cavity (reversing the direction of water flow). Although less efficient, it will provide the fish with adequate oxygen and help prevent water entering the surgical field.

120 An established 150-L aquarium contains African cichlids. The owner complains of lethargy, hiding, and a decreased interest in food in all the fish. Some fish have an increased respiratory rate and effort, and two have died in the past 24 hours. Filtration consists of an external power filter and an undergravel filter with two power heads. Regular water changes are performed, as is weekly testing of water parameters.

Two weeks ago, the tank was medicated for a suspected bacterial fin rot with 20 p.p.m. of chloramphenicol every other day for three treatments, with a 50% water change between each treatment. The owner reports that the fish improved after the treatment.

Water quality parameters are as follows:

Temperature = 27°C (80.6°F)   Nitrite = 3.0 p.p.m.
Ammonia = 2.5 p.p.m.   pH = 8.2

i. What is the likely diagnosis?
ii. What treatments are indicated?

121 i. What organ in this goldfish is affected by the multilobular lesion (**121**)?
ii. What is the probable cause?

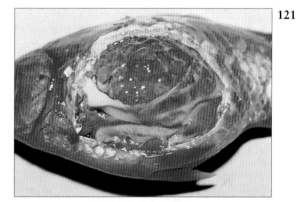

121

122 This melon butterflyfish has obvious skin lesions in the form of multifocal ulcerations (**122a**). The lesions are caused by an external protozoal parasite.
i. What organisms are on your differential list?
ii. How would you confirm your diagnosis?

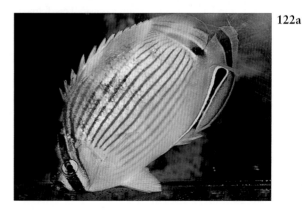

122a

123 This lionfish presented with a raised, irregular cutaneous mass on the right side of its body just below the dorsal fin (**123a, b**). The fish was housed in a 90,000-L aquarium containing numerous lionfish of the same species. Other lionfish in the aquarium appeared normal and the water quality parameters were within normal limits.

i. What are the possible causes of the cutaneous lesion observed on this fish?

ii. How would you manage this case?

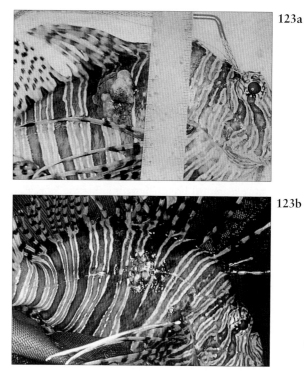

123a

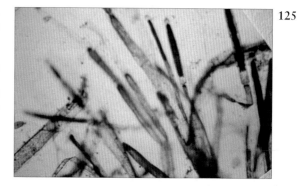

123b

124 You are in a situation where you have diagnosed a bacterial problem in a group of fish by ruling out water quality, parasites, and other problems. You have taken samples for bacterial culture and sensitivity but the results will not be available for at least 48 hours. Name three antibiotic treatment regimens.

125 This organism was observed on a skin scraping taken from a goldfish (**125**).

i. What is it?

ii. What treatment might be given?

iii. What other precautions should be taken before treatment is prescribed?

123 i. The most common cause of cutaneous lesions on a lionfish is an inflammatory response, such as a cutaneous granuloma. Inflammatory lesions can result from infectious agents and noninfectious agents. Another possible cause of this condition would be a cutaneous neoplasm.

ii. After the lionfish was properly anesthetized with MS-222 (100 p.p.m.) the mass was excised using a scalpel blade and the wound was sealed using a drop of cyanoacrylate glue. Cytologic evaluation of an imprint made from the excised tissue revealed a uniform population of epithelial cells with increased cytoplasmic basophilia. There was no evidence of inflammation and an etiology could not be determined. A cytologic diagnosis of epithelial hyperplasia or benign neoplasia was made. The excised mass was placed in 10% neutral buffered formalin and submitted for histopathology. The histopathologic findings indicated an epithelioma, a benign neoplasm. Because the entire mass had been removed during the biopsy procedure, no further treatment was necessary. After two weeks the wound was nearly healed with no evidence of regrowth.

124 *Enrofloxacin:* 5 mg/kg given intramuscularly or intraperitoneally every 48 hours for 15 days; 5 mg/kg orally for 10–14 days or 0.1% in food for 10–14 days; 2.5 p.p.m. as a 5-hour bath repeated every 24 hours for 5–7 days, 50–75% water change between treatments.

Trimethoprim/sulfamethoxazole: 30 mg/kg given intramuscularly or intraperitoneally every 24 hours for 7–10 days; 30 mg/kg orally every 24 hours for 10–14 days or 0.2% in food for 10–14 days; 20 p.p.m. as a 5-hour bath repeated every 24 hours for 5–7 days, 50–75% water change between treatments. Keep water well aerated.

Nitrofurazone: 20 p.p.m. as a 5-hour bath. Repeat daily for 5–7 days. Several soluble forms exist.

There are, of course, numerous possibilities but the three drugs listed have proved effective against many bacterial problems. Sensitivity results can help with antibiotic selection and modification.

125 i. The photograph shows long branched aseptate hyphae characteristic of *Saprolegnia.* This fungus is widespread in fresh and brackish water but does not occur in the marine environment.

ii. The recommended treatments include salt or formalin dips or more prolonged water treatments using mixtures of formalin and malachite green.

iii. Infection is generally regarded as secondary to other underlying factors such as poor management or chronic parasitic infestation. A complete investigation of the problem is therefore essential before initiating treatment. The chemicals used are potentially toxic so their use in the presence of substandard water quality conditions might at best be unsuccessful and at worse cause death of the fish.

126 Albino channel catfish have been purchased and placed in a 209-L display aquarium. The fish are thin and irritable. They constantly rub against decorative objects in the tank. There are tiny tufts (2 mm) of cottony material visible on the dorsal fin rays. A significant amount of fin rot is visible on the caudal fin of all fish.

Water quality parameters from the tank are shown below:

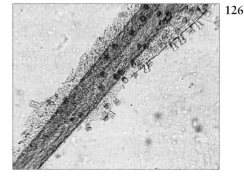

126

Dissolved oxygen: 7.4 p.p.m.
Nitrite: 0 p.p.m.
Temperature: 26°C (78.8°F)
Total alkalinity: 68 p.p.m.
Total ammonia nitrogen: 0.2 p.p.m.
Total hardness: 105 p.p.m.
pH 7.8

Skin biopsies of damaged caudal fins reveal numerous attached ciliates in the genera *Scyphidia* (**126**). Gill biopsies reveal moderate numbers of attached ciliates in the genera *Glossatella* and *Scyphidia*.

i. What is the probable source of infection?
ii. Are other fish in the tank at risk?
iii. What is the best way to manage the problem?
iv. What is the best way to prevent the problem in the future?

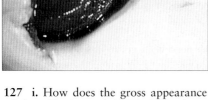

127

127 i. How does the gross appearance of the gill pictured (**127**) differ from normal?
ii. What is the probable cause?
iii. What changes would you expect to see on microscopy?

128 A pond owner calls in the autumn. She complains of several fish deaths in the last three days in a pond which has been trouble free since its installation in the spring.

The pond is roughly 10,000 L, 120 cm deep at its maximum, moderately stocked, and situated close to the house under a large maple tree. A large number of leaves are floating on the surface. Filtration is accomplished by two submersible box filters attached to pumps, each running at 3,000 L/hour. Filter pads are rinsed in pond water every other week.

Water quality parameters are as follows:

Temperature = 17°C (62.6°F)
Total ammonia nitrogen = 1.7 p.p.m.
Nitrite = 1.2 p.p.m.
Dissolved oxygen = 8.0 p.p.m.

What is the likely cause of water quality problems in this pond?

126 i. Sessile protozoans, including *Scyphidia* and *Glossatella*, are most frequently encountered in pond fish. They are particularly common on fish from ponds which are crowded and have a high organic load. Albino catfish fingerlings that are sold through the pet trade frequently originate from channel catfish production facilities, which tend to crowd and heavily stock fish.

ii. The parasites are not likely to cause an immediate problem to tankmates. However, if uncontrolled, the protozoans could accumulate and cause problems in other fish. In addition, if not removed from the catfish, there is a strong likelihood that a secondary bacterial infection will flare up, and depending on the virulence of the bacteria, significant morbidity and mortality could result.

iii. A single treatment with formalin at 25 p.p.m. administered as a bath treatment should control the infestation. If excessive amounts of waste are present in the tank, a thorough cleaning is recommended.

iv. Prevention of commensal protozoans is easier than treating an established infestation. An easy method of minimizing the risk of introducing commensal protozoans is subjecting freshwater fish to a 4–5-minute salt bath (3% solution until they 'roll') before placing them into a display tank. A formalin treatment (up to 250 p.p.m. for 30–60 minutes depending on the species) can also be implemented. Ideally, these prophylactic parasite treatments should be included in the quarantine protocol.

127 i. When normal gills are examined they appear reddish-pink and the separate primary lamellae are clearly visible. In this photograph, the gills are swollen and edematous and have a grayish tinge due to the presence of excessive mucus on the surface. The separate primary lamellae are not clearly distinguishable.

ii. These changes are nonspecific, but are indicative of gill irritation. The causes include irritation by parasites, bacteria, suspended solids, toxins, or metabolic by-products. A fresh gill squash preparation will confirm the presence of excessive mucus and may indicate the presence of protozoan or helminthic parasites. The changes associated with epithelial hyperplasia may be seen on the squash preparation but are more readily seen on stained sections prepared for histopathology.

iii. Examination by microscopy would reveal the following: the secondary lamellae are shortened and rounded and adjacent secondary lamellae are likely to be fused, giving a clubbed appearance. In more advanced cases, the fusion of secondary lamellae becomes complete and there may even be fusion of the primary lamellae resulting in obliteration of the normal gill architecture.

128 A large quantity of leaves decaying on the pond bottom can be a source of water quality problems. Immediate treatment should include daily water changes until the un-ionized ammonia concentration is below 0.1 p.p.m., removal of the decaying plant matter from the pond bottom, and treatment of opportunistic infections as indicated.

Prevention of this problem can be accomplished by covering the pond in the autumn with fine netting or a commercial pond cover, daily skimming of leaves from the pond surface, and/or more frequent water changes.

129 A variety of routes of administration are used to treat pet fish with chemotherapeutants. How would you define the following?
i. Bath.
ii. Dip.
iii. Flush or flow-through.
iv. Indefinite bath.
v. Injectable.
vi. Oral.
vii. Topical.

130 A wholesaler client tells you that he checks the pH of bags of fish which he has received from his suppliers and it is frequently lower than his tank water as well as the shipping water according to the supplier. What is your response?

131 You have just purchased three-dozen golden shiners from a local fish farmer to be used for bait during your weekend fishing trip. When you get home you notice that some of the fish look a little odd (**131a**). You decide to kill one painlessly and examine a squash preparation of the lesions. This is what you find under high magnification (×1,000) (**131b**).

What is your diagnosis, and what should you tell the fish farmer?

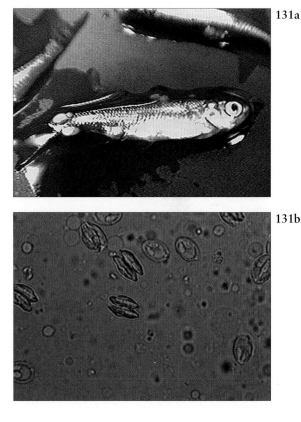

131a

131b

129 i. *Bath:* usually refers to a treatment in which the drug is dissolved in the water in which the fish are swimming. The treatment usually lasts at least 15 minutes and less than 24 hours. Dosage is usually based on volume of water and not fish biomass.

ii. *Dip:* refers to a treatment in which the fish is submerged in a particular solution for between one second and 15 minutes. Water volumes are usually smaller than those of bath treatments.

iii. *Flush or flow-through:* requires constant water flow. Most frequently used in raceways or narrow vats. Medicant is added to inflow area and fish are exposed to drug as it passes over them with the water current. It is similar to the dip procedure except that the fish may not have to be removed from their normal holding area.

iv. *Indefinite bath:* self-explanatory. Medication is added to the tank or pond and usually there is no water change or immediate re-treatment.

v. *Injectable:* medication which is given by injection into the body of the fish with the aid of a hypodermic needle and syringe. Routes may be subcutaneous, intradermal, intramuscular, intravenous, and intraperitoneal.

vi. *Oral:* medication is mixed with the food in order to treat the fish. It is usually done by incorporating drug into a food mixture. For larger fish patients, medication can be placed in a chunk of food and then fed or force fed to the sick fish.

vii. *Topical:* medication is applied directly to the lesion or parasite.

Remember, before using any drug in the water, discontinue any chemical (e.g. carbon) filtration during treatment as this will inactivate the medicant. Adequate aeration is also important during any water treatment.

When antibiotics are used as bath treatments, ideally they should be used daily for seven to ten days. Water changes (at least 50%) should take place between treatments. This protocol is much easier to follow in a home or hospital tank than in a pet store or wholesale facility.

Finally, always perform a biotest with one or two animals when working with unfamiliar drugs, water, or species to determine if the fish will tolerate the treatment.

130 You explain some of the biochemistry occurring within the shipping bag. Heavy loads of fish will excrete large amounts of carbon dioxide. This will react with the water to form carbonic acid, which will dissociate, releasing hydrogen ions into the water. These hydrogen ions will react with the alkalinity in the water, reducing the buffering capacity, and simultaneously lowering the pH. A bag which may have started out with a pH of 8.0 could easily, after 12–24 hours of shipping, have a pH of 7.0 because of this CO_2 build-up. Additionally, the accumulation of organic acids and heterotrophic bacterial activity will also contribute to this pH reduction.

131 This animal was severely infected with myxosporidian parasites. You would want to inform the farmer of this finding and recommend that he examine fish from his breeding stock. Because this disease is not treatable and will probably reduce his production, you would advise that infected stocks should be culled and the tanks disinfected with a bleach solution if this is economically and physically possible.

132 A freshwater angelfish breeder is experiencing difficulty raising fry. The number of eggs laid by his broodstock has decreased over the past few months, with only a 70% hatching success. Of the fry that do hatch, only about 40% survive to the swim-up stage. Water quality in a typical hatching jar is shown below:

Dissolved oxygen: 7.5 p.p.m.
Total ammonia nitrogen: 1.4 p.p.m.
Temperature: 26°C (78.8°F)
pH: 7.2
Total alkalinity: 140 p.p.m.
Nitrite: 0 p.p.m.
Total hardness: 120 p.p.m.

Examination of broodstock reveals small numbers of motile flagellates in the intestinal tract. Examination of eggs and fry with light microscopy reveals large numbers of flagellated protozoans on the external surface of the eggs, and internally and externally in the fry.
i. What is the most likely cause of poor egg quality, hatch rate, and fry survival?
ii. What is the most likely source of infection?
iii. What do you recommend to correct the problem?

133 Several deaths have occurred in a pond that is served by this single-chamber biologic filter which contains an expanded clay gravel media. The chamber has been drained for inspection (**133**).
i. What problem has developed in this filter chamber?
ii. What solution would you recommend?

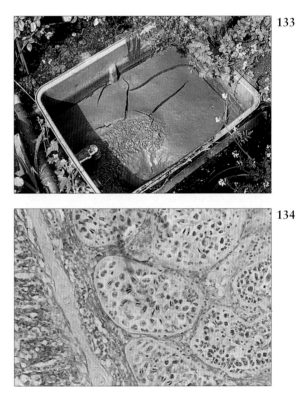
133

134 This slide from the gill of a koi carp has been stained with Giemsa stain (**134**).
i. What characteristic structures are visible?
ii. What is the organism? Describe its life cycle.

134

132 i. *Spironucleus* is a diplomonad flagellate (10–20 μm) which is frequently found in the intestinal tract of angelfish (**132**). They are occasionally found in the intestine of dying fry. Whether or not they are present on the external surface of fry is uncertain. These flagellates are so small that a slide could be easily contaminated with gut contents, giving the impression of external infection.

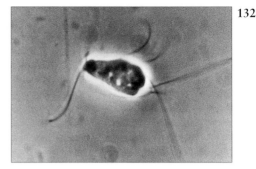

ii. The most likely source of *Spironucleus* in fry is infected broodstock. The apparent level of infection in adults may not be indicative of the level of infection on eggs or in fry. Poor sanitation appears to exacerbate the problem in eggs and fry.

iii. Broodstock of species that are highly susceptible to *Spironucleus* should be treated prophylactically with a metronidazole-medicated food (50 mg/kg fish) every 2–4 months. Species of particular concern include angelfish, discus, oscars, African cichlids, and gouramis. Infected eggs or fry can be treated with a metronidazole bath (at 6 p.p.m.) every other day for three treatments. Particular attention should be paid to sanitation. Dead eggs, fry, and uneaten food should be removed from the environment promptly.

133 i. There is a heavy accumulation of detritus and dead algae which has caused the filter medium to become blocked. This has resulted in inefficient removal of metabolic wastes with subsequent deterioration of water quality (a rise in ammonia and nitrite levels).

ii. The filter should be cleaned more frequently to remove this organic matter. A less labor-intensive option is to add a separate settlement reservoir (primary chamber) to this gravel chamber. Water from the pond should be pumped into the primary chamber to allow removal of the suspended solids before the water enters the gravel filter media. Cleaning the sediment from the settlement chamber is still required but is facilitated by a drain tap at the bottom of the chamber.

134 i. The gross lesions of this condition appear as small, discrete, smooth, rounded nodules on the gill. The color is similar to that of the surrounding gill tissue with no apparent hyperemia or inflammation.

The section stained with Giemsa indicates the distinct polar bodies characteristic of the myxozoan parasite, *Henneguya koi*.

ii. *Henneguya koi* is an intracellular parasite, which invades target cells and develops into a pseudocyst, producing large numbers of spores. Spores are normally released when the fish dies, although they can be released earlier if pseudocysts situated on the epithelial surface rupture. Usually only individual fish are affected. There is no treatment, although it is wise to remove the affected fish to avoid spread to others.

135 i. What particular problem do marine fish face with regard to their osmoregulation?
ii. What physiologic mechanisms are in place to address this problem?

136 A 75-L aquarium with undergravel filtration contains two 10-cm pearl cichlids, a 12-cm *Plecostomus*, a 12-cm striped shovelnose catfish, and two 10-cm jewel cichlids. Until one week before presentation, there had been no problems with disease, mortality, or water quality. Two weeks ago, the two jewel cichlids were added after a four-week quarantine. In the past week, the fish have become progressively more lethargic and inappetent, spending more time hiding or resting on the bottom. In the past day, the catfish has developed a generalized whitish appearance to its body.

Water quality parameters are as follows:

Temperature: 28°C (82.4°F)
pH: 7.2
Total ammonia nitrogen: 2.0 p.p.m.
Nitrite: 1.5 p.p.m.

i. What is the likely diagnosis?
ii. How should the immediate problem be controlled?
iii. What long-term options are there for preventing recurrence while retaining this population of fish?

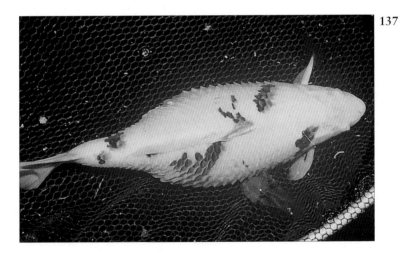

137

137 i. What clinical feature is seen affecting the skin of this koi (137)?
ii. Suggest some causes for this condition.

135 i. The body fluids of marine fish are hypotonic to their environment, the concentrations being about 25–30% of seawater. As a result of diffusion and osmosis, there is a tendency for water to leave the fish's body and for salts to enter. It is essential for the normal physiologic processes of the fish that the concentrations of body fluids are controlled within narrow limits.

ii. The factors involved in the control of the concentrations of the body fluids of marine fish are listed: (A) Limitation of the overall permeable surface area. The structure of the normal skin with its mucus layer ensures that the skin surface remains impermeable. Thus the surface area available for the exchange of water is reduced to that of the gill, and to a lesser extent the bowel. This factor is important in those diseases in which the skin surface becomes ulcerated. (B) The uptake of water from the gastrointestinal tract. Marine fish continually drink saltwater at a rate of about 0.5% of body weight per hour. This in turn results in the absorption of sodium and chloride ions through the bowel. (C) Excretory processes within the kidney. The urine of marine fish is more concentrated than that of freshwater fish. The maximum concentration achieved can only be that of the body fluids and so this does not represent a net excretion of salts. Magnesium and sulphate ions are excreted in the urine. (D) Excretory processes in the gill. The principal agents of salt excretion are the chloride cells situated within the gill epithelium. This is an active process in which sodium and chloride ions are excreted, producing localized areas of a high concentration of salt with resultant local diffusion gradients.

136 i. It is likely that the problems are due to overstocking. The existing filtration, if designed for a 75-L tank, is probably inadequate to process the nitrogenous wastes produced by this population of fish.

ii. Immediate therapy should be aimed at lowering the levels of nitrogenous toxins by multiple partial water changes and the addition of zeolite if desired, addition of NaCl at 500 p.p.m., and decreasing the stocking density.

iii. Options for increasing allowable stocking density include: (A) Increasing the surface area for bacterial growth by using a finer filter medium, adding more filter medium, or adding additional filtration. (B) Increasing the water flow rate over the existing filter substrate by using a pump with a higher LPH (liters per hour) rating or adding power heads to an undergravel filter. (C) Increasing the frequency of water changes. (D) Increasing the oxygenation of the water being filtered.

137 i. Scale edema and 'dropsy' produces this characteristic 'pine cone' appearance.

ii. Dropsy can result from infection or neoplasia. The subsequent tissue damage in the skin, gills, heart, liver, or kidneys produces a failure of osmoregulation and development of edema and/or ascites. Retrobulbar accumulation of tissue fluid may or may not produce exophthalmia which may be unilateral or bilateral. In this case the fish had a large hepatic tumor.

138 What kind of everyday household products might interfere with the water quality of a tank or pond?

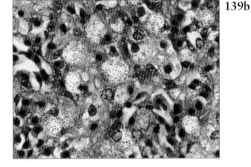

39a

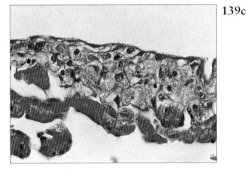

139b

139 This is a Giemsa-stained blood film from a blue-eyed plecostomus (**139a**). The pictured cell is a monocyte containing numerous basophilic granules in the cytoplasm. From the history provided, you know that several leeches were removed from the fish by the wholesaler that owns this fish. Several fish from a population of 20 have died and another six are debilitated. On necropsy, histopathology reveals similar large accumulations of these obligate intracytoplasmic organisms in the spleen (**139b**), kidney, and heart (epicardium) (**139c**).

139c

i. What is your list of differentials?
ii. How would you go about pursuing a definitive diagnosis?
iii. What are the clinical implications of this condition?

140 A gill squash preparation is frequently used to investigate the presence of gill disease (**140**).

What is the procedure for obtaining a gill squash?

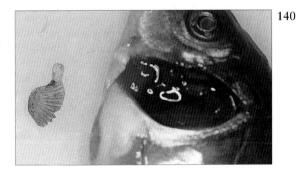

140

138 Indoors, spray furniture polish used on the outside and top cover of a tank can cause problems to fish. Any cleaning fluids on or around a tank should be avoided. Ordinary clean water should eliminate any irritating dirty marks on a tank. Tobacco smoke has potentially deleterious effects. Insecticides and other pesticides (flea and tick bombs) should also be avoided in the presence of an aquarium. If these compounds must be used and the fish cannot be moved, disconnect the air source for several hours and cover the aquarium with a towel or sheet. Sudden changes in light are not helpful to the well-being of fish: they do not have eyelids and cannot close their eyes when confronted with bright lights. Outdoor ponds may suffer from chemical pollution caused by gardeners spilling chemicals. Leaching of soil containing these chemicals might occur in certain circumstances. In all of these cases, partial water changes and elimination of the contaminant will help to rectify the situation.

139 i. Rickettsia-like organisms, intracellular hemoparasites, intracellular bacteria.
ii. Assuming adequate available funding, transmission electron microscopy will reveal the ultrastructure of these granules (**139d**). The electron micrograph pictured here shows organisms with the characteristic features of a rickettsia. The shape, size, and triple membrane are consistent with rickettsia-like organisms found

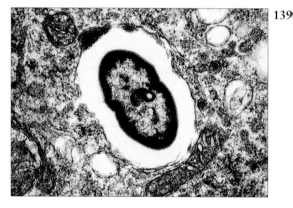
139

in blue-eyed plecos and other fish, including salmonids.
iii. Several reports have linked rickettsia-like organisms with clinical disease in fish. Proper quarantine practices combined with antibiotic therapy appropriate for rickettsia is warranted.

140 A small amount (no more than a 0.5 cm cube) of the soft gill tissue is obtained from a freshly dead fish. This tissue is spread out on a microscope slide in a drop of water (preferably water from the pond or tank from which the fish was taken: tap or distilled water may destroy any parasites present) and a cover slip applied. The preparation should be examined under the microscope. Standard optics should be sufficient to visualize parasites, fungal infection, and irritant particulate matter. Oil immersion may be necessary to visualize bacterial gill disease. It is possible to obtain a gill preparation from an anesthetized fish by carefully raising the operculum and using a fine pair of scissors to remove the distal 3–4 mm of three to six primary gill lamellae.

141 A recently imported group of snakeheads are losing weight and appear generally unthrifty. Snakeheads are aggressive, freshwater tropical fish that are native to Asia. Water quality parameters are within normal limits and gill, skin, and fin biopsies are unremarkable. The picture (**141a**) is from a direct fecal examination.

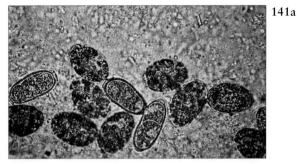

141a

i. What types of ova are present?
ii. How would you manage this problem?

142 You are in a situation where you have diagnosed a protozoal ectoparasitic problem in a group of fish. The fish are sick and need immediate treatment. You are managing the water quality adequately and are ready to begin treatment.

Name three parasiticide treatment regimens.

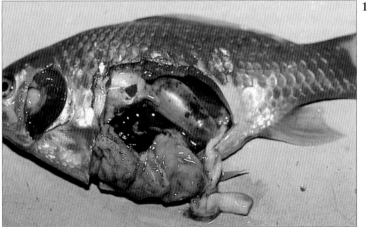

143

143 i. What is the principal lesion seen in the photograph (**143**)?
ii. What infectious agents might be involved?

141b

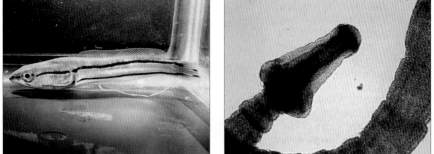

141

141 i. Nematode as well as cestode eggs are present.
ii. A 2.0 p.p.m. praziquantel treatment for three hours caused the fish to expel many intact cestodes. A mature cestode can be seen trailing from the vent of this snakehead (**141b**). In general, most ornamental fish will tolerate a praziquantel bath of between 2.0 and 10.0 p.p.m. for up to six hours. The nematode infection can be treated with a levamisole bath of 2.0 p.p.m. for 24 hours. Both of these treatments should be repeated in 14–21 days. The microscopic view of the cestode clearly shows the scolex and proglottids (**141c**). This cestode probably belongs in the genus *Circumonocobothrium*.

142 Ectoparasitic protozoans must be treated with a dip or bath. *Salt water:* many freshwater species will tolerate a 4–5-minute dip in full-strength (30–35 g/L) salt water. Marine fish can be placed in a freshwater dip for 4–5 minutes. Aerate well and monitor very closely. Certain smaller fish may not survive this treatment. If possible, test treatment on one fish first. *Formaldehyde:* at 10–20 p.p.m. for 12–24 hours followed by a 50% water change. Encysted parasites like 'Ich' and *Cryptocaryon* will require several treatments. Always change water between treatments and aerate the treatment water well because formalin decreases the amount of oxygen available to the fish. *Metronidazole:* as a bath treatment it will kill some external flagellates, at 10 p.p.m. every 24 hours for three consecutive days, water changes between treatments.

143 i. The picture shows a gross postmortem examination of a koi carp with the left abdominal wall removed. The surface of the bowel has a number of small petechial hemorrhages. Large hemorrhages are present on the posterior portion of the swim bladder.
ii. These changes are consistent with a generalized septicemia, viremia, or toxemia, and sampling for bacteriology and histopathology would be necessary to make a specific diagnosis. One viral agent, swim-bladder inflammation (SBI) virus, a rhabdovirus, specifically affects this organ causing degenerative changes with congestion, hemorrhage, and sloughing of the necrotic epithelium into the lumen. This particular virus usually affects cyprinids and is sometimes described as a component of the carp dropsy syndrome. It is very similar to spring viremia of carp (SVC), although SVC is thought to be a distinct entity.

144 These rapidly spinning ciliated organisms were seen on the examination of a skin scrape (×100) (**144a**).
i. Name the organism.
ii. How is a skin scraping prepared?

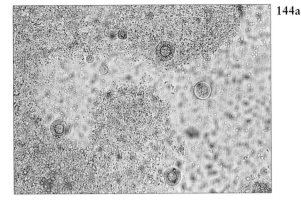

144a

145 i. What is this organism (**145**)?
ii. What clue does the picture reveal regarding its life cycle?
iii. Does this have clinical significance?

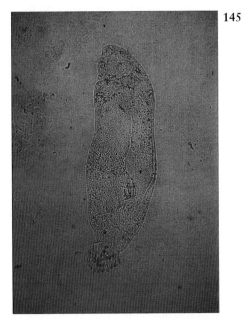

145

146 You are in a situation where you have diagnosed an ectoparasitic monogenean problem in a group of fish. The fish are quite sick and in need of immediate treatment. You are managing the water quality adequately and are ready to begin treatment.
    Name three parasiticide treatment regimens.

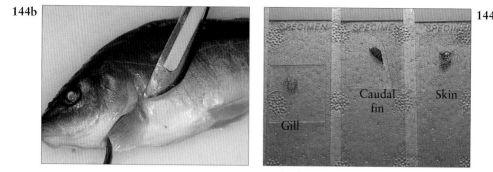

144 i. *Trichodina*, a ciliated protozoan parasite which is a common cause of skin and gill disease in ornamental fish.
ii. A skin scrape is prepared by obtaining a small quantity of mucus from the skin surface of a freshly dead or anesthetized fish (**144b**). Areas of predilection for skin parasites are those adjacent to the fins and it is a good approach to obtain material from these sites. The mucus is suspended in a small quantity of water on a microscope slide (preferably pond or tank water from which the fish was taken; tap or distilled water may destroy the parasites), a cover slip applied, and the preparation examined under the microscope (×40 magnification should be sufficient to visualize most parasites). The second picture shows prepared gill, fin, and skin biopsies (**144c**).

145 i. The photomicrograph is of *Gyrodactylus,* a freshwater monogenean skin fluke. The characteristic features enabling it to be recognized from *Dactylogyrus* (the gill fluke) are the paired hooks with which it anchors to the skin and the lack of eye spots characteristic of *Dactylogyrus*.
ii. This fluke has a direct ovoviviperous life cycle and careful examination of the photograph will reveal the presence of an embryonated larva with its own set of hooks. This allows for rapid, temperature-dependent reproduction.
iii. The nature of the life cycle means that a single treatment may be sufficient to control the infestation. This is different from the oviparous species in which the eggs are resistant to treatment, allowing re-infestation to occur. In the latter case, several parasiticide treatments may be required.

146 *Praziquantel:* 5–10 p.p.m. as a 3–6-hour bath, repeat in seven days. Place fish in a treatment tank if possible and aerate the water well. Some marine species may be sensitive to praziquantel. The aquarium may still be contaminated so treated fish should be moved to a new aquarium if possible. Praziquantel may not kill all species of monogeneans. This treatment will kill most internal cestodes. *Saltwater/freshwater dips:* may be effective against some parasites. Marine fish can be placed in a freshwater dip for 4–5 minutes and freshwater fish placed in saltwater (35 p.p.t. salt) for 4–5 minutes. *Acetic acid:* 2 ml glacial acetic acid/L water as a 30–45-second dip is safe for goldfish but smaller tropical fish may not tolerate this treatment.

147 What factors need to be considered when selecting a therapeutic protocol for the treatment of bacterial ulcers in pond fish (**147**)?

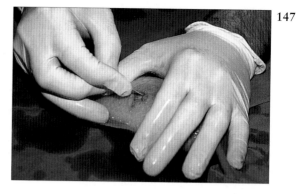

148 i. What is this tissue (**148**)?
ii. What are the black foci at the periphery of this organ?

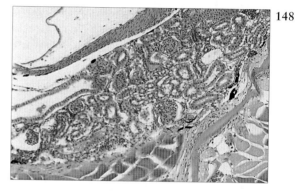

149 You are presented with a problem in which a number of fish are showing rapid swimming motions and are rubbing against rocks in the pond. The colors of some of the fish have become dull (**149**).
i. What would be your provisional list of differentials?
ii. How would you go about investigating the problem?

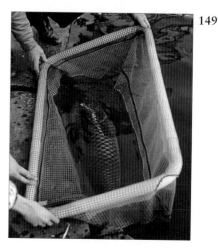

147 Bacterial ulcers in pond fish may result from an infected wound but are commonly a sequela to septicemia. Often the disease outbreak results from a stress factor such as water quality problems or parasitism, and it is important to correct these problems as part of the overall therapeutic program.

Ulcer treatment protocol:

- Parenteral antibiotics. Ideally the choice should be based on specific identification and culture and sensitivity tests. In practice, however, an educated guess may be made so that therapy can be started while the tests are progressing. Once the results are known, the treatment can be modified as appropriate. If a large number of fish are affected, it is most practical to give the antibiotic in the food. In cases where the fish are not eating, or if only a small number are affected, administration of the antibiotic by injection is most practical.
- Topical preparations. Under sedation or anesthesia, the ulcer should be thoroughly debrided to remove all necrotic material. Antiseptics such as povidone iodine can be applied directly to the ulcerated surface. Some clinicians favor the use of topical antibiotic sprays or they may locally infiltrate the lesion with an antibiotic injection.
- Fluid balance. An important consideration when dealing with ulcers is that the normal waterproof coating of the fish has been breached, allowing disruption of the fish's fluid balance mechanisms. It is therefore important to attempt to repair this by applying a layer of a polybasic barrier cream over the topical treatments discussed above. In addition, it is common practice in cold-water ponds to add salt to the water to reduce the concentration gradient across the ulcer.

148 i. Caudal or tail kidney. Identifiable by the numerous tubules and glomeruli. These structures are absent in the hematopoietic cranial or head kidney.
ii. Melanin. A normal finding.

149 i. The dullness of the coloration is caused by an excessive layer of mucus on the skin. This, together with the behavioral signs described, are the result of skin irritation. This can be caused by parasitic infestation, chemical irritants and toxins, or by suspended solids in the water.
ii. The routine measurement of water quality parameters would indicate whether the cause was related to metabolic toxins such as ammonia or nitrite. Direct observation of the water would allow assessment of the level of suspended solids.

Large parasites, such as leeches, *Lernaea,* and *Argulus,* are visible to the naked eye. However, the condition is more often associated with microscopic parasites that can easily be identified on fresh skin scrapings. This is preferably taken from an unanesthetized fish since the anesthetic agents may cause the parasites to fall off the fish.

The common parasites identified on such scrapings are skin flukes (*Gyrodactylus*) and gill flukes (*Dactylogyrus*), as well as a large range of protozoan parasites (including *Ichthyophthirius, Chilodonella,* and *Trichodina*).

150 This oranda goldfish presented with a large mass just dorsal to the lateral line and ventral to the dorsal fin (**150a**). The plan was to surgically remove the mass and submit it for histopathologic evaluation. What noninvasive method would you use to define the mass further and determine whether or not it has involved the vertebral column?

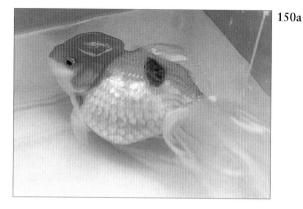

151 i. What lesion is visible in this photomicrograph (**151**)?
ii. What is its clinical significance?

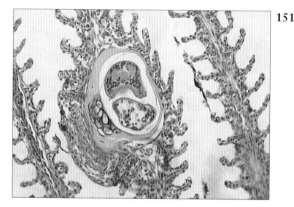

152 This squirrelfish has unilateral exophthalmia which slowly evolved over the last week (**152a**).
i. What is the layman's term for this clinical syndrome?
ii. What causes would be included on your differential list?
iii. What diagnostic tests would you perform to determine the cause of the problem?

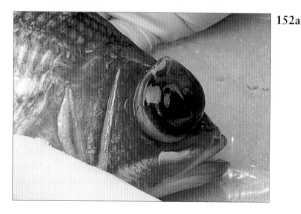

150 A lateral radiograph showed the mass to be well isolated
above the vertebral column with
no apparent metastasis to deep-
er tissues (150b). Other features
to note in this radiograph are
the otoliths (ear stones), pharyngeal teeth, bilobed swim bladder, and caudal kidney which
can be seen just dorsal to the
center of the swim bladder and
ventral to the spine.

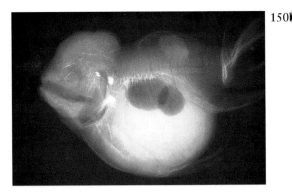

151 i. The photograph shows a section of a platy's gill stained with hematoxylin and
eosin. It shows a cross-section of a metazoan parasite that is encapsulated within the
tissues of the gill. The organism is a metacercaria of a dignenean trematode. It is encapsulated within the gill tissue. These parasites have a complex life cycle in which cer-
cariae are released from an invertebrate (commonly a gastropod mollusc) and penetrate
the tissues of a second intermediate host (the fish). The life cycle continues when the
larvae enter the primary or definitive host (usually a higher vertebrate) when living or
dead fish are ingested.
ii. This condition does not pose a risk to other fish in the same community tank and
only becomes clinically significant when large numbers of the metacercaria are present.

152 i. The common name for this syndrome is 'pop
eye disease.'
ii. The most common causes for this condition are a
retrobulbar mass (neoplasia, bacterial, or fungal
granuloma), retrobulbar or intraocular gas, and
pseudobranch pathophysiology.
iii. The eye should be examined thoroughly using
ophthalmic instruments like this slit lamp device
(152b). Intraocular gas in the anterior chamber can
help differentiate whether the problem is intraocular
or retrobulbar. A transcorneal intraocular aspirate
can be taken at the limbus using a 27-gauge needle
attached to a tuberculin syringe. This technique not
only relieves intraocular pressure but it also produces
a sterile sample for microbiologic culture. Aspiration
of the retrobulbar chamber can be performed for cytology or culture and can be handled in a similar

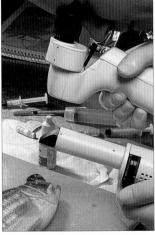

manner to the intraocular technique. A small amount of sterile saline can be introduced
into the chamber through the periocular skin and collected with the same needle by
inverting the fish and aspirating at the most dependent portion of the conjunctiva.

153 With regard to the squirrelfish in **152**, how would you treat the problem?

154 A home aquarist with a fairly extensive collection of saltwater tropical fish phones your practice informing you of an emergency situation with one of his juvenile barracudas. He collected the animals last week and placed them on display in a large circular tank in the center of his living room. All three fish appeared healthy an hour ago but now one is lying on its side on the bottom of the tank and the caudal two-thirds of its body is darker than its head. He is worried that the barracudas have some infectious disease and now he has introduced it to his prize display tank.

What is the most likely diagnosis of this animal's problem. and what should you advise the owner to do?

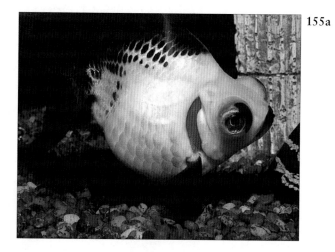

155a

155 This recently purchased fancy goldfish presents because of what the owner describes as a very red gill (**155a**). She did not notice the condition when she purchased the fish.

What will your diagnostic work-up consist of?

153 (A) Rule out and if appropriate resolve any environmental gas supersaturation problem. (B) Protect the eye from trauma by removing unessential aquarium furniture and covering the sides of the tank to prevent excitation of the fish. (C) If gas-producing bacteria are cultured, medicate appropriately and relieve gas pressure periodically through aspiration. (D) For those species which have a pseudobranch, gas production due to pseudobranch pathophysiology is usually identified through a process of elimination. Carbonic anhydrase inhibitors such as acetazolamide can be used but are difficult to dose correctly. Carbonic anhydrase enzymes also control gas bladder pressure in physoclystous fish and the use of carbonic anhydrase inhibitors can result in buoyancy problems. Unilateral pseudobranchectomy has relieved exophthalmic lesions refractory to medical treatment. The pseudobranch can be cauterized in small fish and can be ablated surgically in larger fish after efferent and afferent vessels are ligated Anatomy of the pseudobranch varies greatly between species.

154 The animal has a spinal fracture (**154**). Recently wild-caught barracudas have the tendency to bolt if they are frightened and this one could have easily collided with the tank wall. You should strongly remind the owner that the most important factor in main-

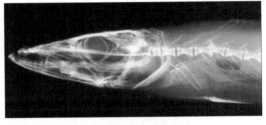

154

taining his fish collection's health is a rigid quarantine program. At the very least the animals should have been housed away from his long-standing collection for 30 days.

155 Examine the other opercu-lum (**155b**). It is normal. This fish is missing part of its right operculum but the underlying gill tissue on the affected side appears grossly unremarkable.

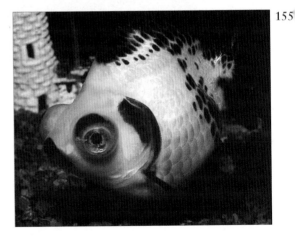

155

156 With regard to the goldfish in **155**, what will you tell the owner about the fish's prognosis?

157 A large garden pond (10 × 20 m) has been stocked with goldfish and large albino channel catfish. The pond was designed to meander through a part of the garden that borders a low lying area with a creek. The pond owner is well educated about pond management and has maintained detailed records of fish stocked including stocking dates, species, size, and total number. Many of the goldfish have pet names and are easily recognized by their individual markings. No dead or dying animals have ever been observed. Despite all of the care taken, fish seem to 'disappear' sporadically from the pond. Although this is most obvious when individually named fish cannot be found, it seems that the number of albino catfish has decreased dramatically over the past few weeks.
i. Based on the narrative provided, what would be a plausible explanation for the complaint?
ii. How would you confirm your suspicion?
iii. What steps could be taken to remedy the problem?

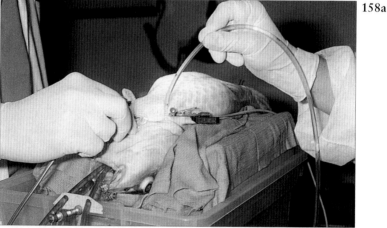

158a

158 You are preparing a koi for surgery to remove an abdominal mass. Your anesthetic protocol is established and you plan on a mid-ventral incision with the fish in dorsal recumbency (**158a**).
i. How will you monitor the fish while it is anesthetized?
ii. How will you prepare the incision site?

156 The most likely cause of this condition is either traumatic or congenital. Fish with this problem are usually culled at the wholesale level or sold at a reduced price. The gill tissue is somewhat more vulnerable without the protective operculum, but if the husbandry is adequate, the problem is primarily aesthetic.

157 i. Any time animals disappear with no history of a fish kill, predation should be suspected. The location of the pond, adjacent to a low lying area and creek, is particularly suspicious. Otters are voracious predators which often gain access to a fish farm or pond from an adjacent creek. In certain parts of the southern USA, alligators can also be serious predators, and they often live in

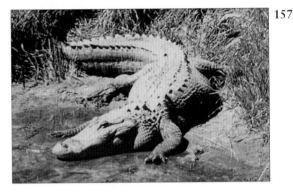
157

low swampy areas, including creeks and lakes (**157**). Aquatic snakes also readily consume pond fish when they can catch them.

ii. In Florida, alligators are common and there is a possibility of one being in the vicinity of a pond adjacent to a lowland (or swampy) area. To confirm the presence of alligators, it is best to walk around the entire pond looking for their tracks. They have characteristic feet, and the mark left by their tail is usually discernible as well.

iii. If alligator tracks are discovered, an effective method of discouraging them from approaching the pond is to place electric wire around the periphery at a height of about 3–6 cm.

158 i. Opercular movement is a good indicator of life, but in cases where the fish needs to be very deep, opercular movements may cease. Electrocardiography is an option, with leads placed at the base of each pectoral fin and one near the vent. The alligator clips can be attached to small needles placed in the skin.

ii. A clear sterile surgical drape should be used and the scales

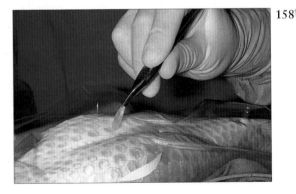
158

removed along the planned incision line (**158b**). The skin can be treated carefully with a pre-surgical antiseptic, although this may not be necessary.

159 With regard to the koi in **158**, how will you manage the case post-operatively?

160 An African cichlid breeder has experienced chronic, low-level mortality in certain groups of fish. Fish are housed in 950-L vats on a flow-through system. Water exchange occurs every 60–90 minutes and stocking densities are moderate to heavy. Severe infestations with *Trichodina* are frequently found on gills or skin of unthrifty and dying fish (**160a, b**). Repeated treatment with formalin at 25 p.p.m. has slowed mortality but has not eliminated the problem. Water quality parameters from a representative vat are listed below:

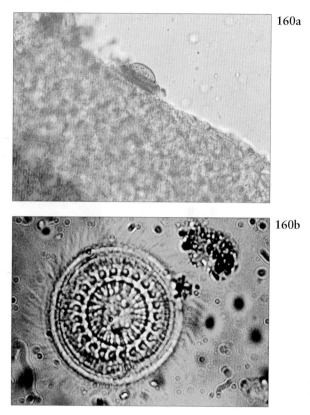

160a

160b

Dissolved oxygen: 6 p.p.m.
Total ammonia: 2 p.p.m.
Temperature: 30°C (86°F)
pH: 8.2
Total alkalinity: 220 p.p.m.
Toxic ammonia: 0.2 p.p.m.
Total hardness: 280 p.p.m.
Nitrite: 0.5 p.p.m.

i. What factors are likely to contribute to a chronic *Trichodina* problem?
ii. In general, what treatment should be recommended for *Trichodina*?
iii. What steps may need to be taken to correct the situation described above?

159 The mass turned out to be an ovarian granulosa-theca cell tumor and it was removed uneventfully (159a). The skin was closed with nonabsorbable nylon suture and air was aspirated from the abdominal compartment following surgical closure (159b). Note the use of an extra plastic tube to provide fresh water to the gills (two tubes providing water flow are in the mouth of the fish). Enrofloxacin was administered intramuscularly at a dose of 10 mg/kg every 48 hours for ten days. This fish recovered and was doing well five months after surgery.

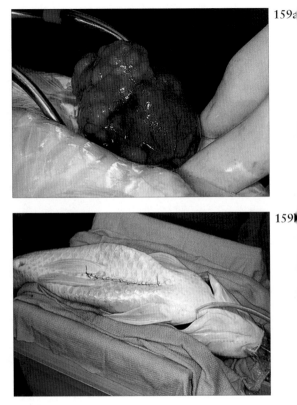

159a

159b

160 i. *Trichodina* is a motile, ciliated protozoan and a common gill and skin parasite on fish. This parasite thrives under conditions of crowding, heavy feeding, and high organic load. Warm temperatures may also exacerbate *Trichodina* problems.

ii. In general, any of the chemicals which are effective against external protozoans should be efficacious against *Trichodina*. The parasite's direct life cycle dictates that one treatment should be adequate. Examples of efficacious chemicals include formalin, copper sulfate, potassium permanganate, or salt.

iii. In the situation described, thorough cleaning of the environment will be necessary, including removal of all organic debris. Stocking rate, feeding rate, and water exchange rate may need to be adjusted to avoid accumulation of excessive organic debris in the future. Once the environment is clean, a single treatment with one of the chemicals listed above should result in decreased mortality and improved condition of the fish.

161 i. What lesion is present on the eye of this goldfish (161)?
ii. What course of action is required?

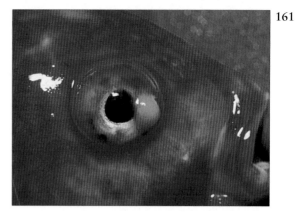

161

162 A group of goldfish were purchased. Because construction of their pond had not been completed, the owner elected to house them in galvanized steel tanks that he borrowed from a friend. After three days the fish began to die. Water quality parameters were as follows:

Dissolved oxygen: 7.0 p.p.m.
Total ammonia nitrogen: 3.0 p.p.m.
Temperature: 26°C (78.8°F)
Nitrite: 0.5 p.p.m.

Total alkalinity: 51 p.p.m.
pH: 8.2
Total hardness: 68 p.p.m.
Chloride: 155 p.p.m.

A fish that had just died was collected by the owner and brought in for necropsy. Gill and skin biopsies were negative. A bacterial culture taken from the posterior kidney showed no growth after 48 hours at 25°C (77°F).
i. Which heavy metal can leach from galvanized steel and cause mortality in fish?
ii. How would you confirm your diagnosis?
iii. How would water quality parameters affect the situation?

163 This kohaku koi presented for a laceration just caudal to the head. The owner suspected a bird strike (163a).

How would you manage this wound?

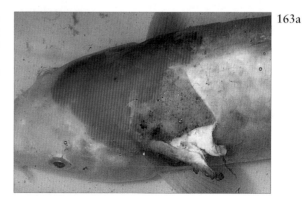

163a

161 i. A fibroma.

ii. Removal of these tumors are rarely without complication since they may involve the full thickness of the cornea. The tumors are usually benign, but may progress slowly and with time may cover most of the cornea. In the absence of ulceration and secondary infection, it is advised that these tumors are left untreated since the fish are often clinically unaffected.

162 i. Zinc toxicity is commonly associated with fish mortality after housing in a galvanized steel tank.

ii. When a toxin is suspected, efforts should be made to confirm the presence of the suspect contaminant in the environment and in tissue of affected fish. State veterinary diagnostic laboratories are usually able to perform these assays at a reasonable cost. In the situation described, a water sample from the tank should be frozen in an inert plastic bottle. A few freshly dead or moribund fish should be frozen in a plastic bag. These samples should then be submitted to the appropriate laboratory for analysis.

iii. Toxicity of zinc to fish varies dramatically between different species of fish and water quality parameters. A number of studies have reported 96-h LC50 data in the range of 0.87–40.90 p.p.m. Zn^{2+} in water. In general, zinc toxicity increases as water temperature and pH increase, and total hardness decreases.

163 Because the wound is obviously contaminated with dirt and debris, the tissues should be flushed with saline, clean water, or a dilute antiseptic. In this case, the fish was anesthetized with tricaine methanesulfonate and the wound was cleaned with dilute chlorhexidine solution. The skin flap was sutured with 4-0 absorbable suture material in a simple interrupted pattern (**163b**). The wound healed uneventfully with very little scarring.

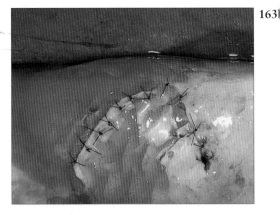

163b

164 The owner of a 135-L community tank reports that her neon tetras have been disappearing slowly over the past week. She suspects predation as the cause of the disappearance.

Which of the following fish is most likely to prey on small fish such as tetras?
A Gold gourami.
B Angelfish.
C Pictus catfish.
D Cory catfish.

165 This green terror cichlid presented with pale white to gray nodular lesions on the pectoral fins, opercula, and caudal fin (**165a**). The fish is eating and appears to be strong. Water quality parameters are within normal limits. No other fish are affected.
i. What conditions are on your differential list?
ii. How would you confirm a diagnosis?
iii. How would you manage this problem?

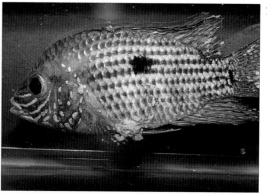

165a

166 This leopard shark was found dead in a 150,000-L outdoor aquarium in the southeastern USA (**166**). The aquarium consisted of a round concrete pool buried in the ground with the water surface approximately 30 cm below the ground level. Other sharks and bony fish in the aquarium appeared healthy. A gross necropsy revealed a hemorrhagic gastritis and a large intact toad was found in the stomach.

What is the most probable cause of death in this shark?

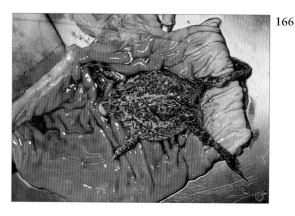

166

109

164 C. *Pimelodus*, even when relatively small, have mouths large enough to engulf neon tetras (164). They are generally well tolerated as community fish, but should not be housed with fish much smaller than themselves.

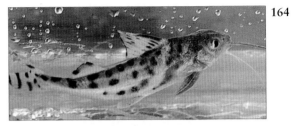

164

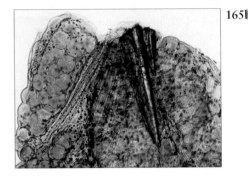

165I

165 i. Lymphocystis disease, neoplasia, fungal infection, and protozoal disease (e.g. *Heteropolaria*).
ii. The diagnosis is made by taking a biopsy of the lesion and examining a wet mount under the light microscope. This is a case of lymphocystis disease. The infection causes a marked hypertrophy of the dermal connective tissue cells. Individual cells are frequently visible to the naked eye. Clusters of round cells of various size (hypertrophied fibroblasts) will indicate a diagnosis of lymphocystis disease (165b). Diagnosis can be confirmed with histology and/or electron microscopy. This is the most common viral disease of ornamental fish. The disease is caused by an iridovirus and has been identified in over 100 species of fish. Transmission is probably horizontal, although not all fish exposed will contract the disease. Viral particles can survive for at least several days in the water and sub-clinical carriers probably exist. Lymphocystis disease is frequently self-limiting, although affected fish should be isolated.
iii. Environmental stresses should be removed. Affected fish should be isolated for at least six weeks. If practical, lesions can be surgically removed and the fish monitored for secondary bacterial infections.

166 Apparently, the toad fell into the open aquarium where it had easy access and was eaten by the shark. The giant tropical toad, *Bufo marinus*, was introduced to the southeastern USA in the early 1970s as a method to control undesirable insects. All toads and especially this species produce a toxic substance from their parotid glands. The thick, cream-colored toxic secretion is easily expressed from pinhole openings on the skin overlying the parotid glands. Mortality rates of dogs in the southeastern USA exposed to oral contact with the toxins from *Bufo marinus* approach 100%. The bufotoxins secreted from the parotid glands have a digitalis-like effect, resulting in ventricular fibrillation in mammals. Other compounds found in the toxic secretions include epinephrine, cholesterol, ergosterol, and 5-hydroxytryptamine. Orally ingested bufotoxins in sharks can result in acute death and a hemorrhagic gastritis.

167 A juvenile, black grouper approximately six years old presents with acute anorexia, lethargy and a slight skin darkening over the caudal one-third of its body. The fish is a three-year resident of a 240,000-L community Atlantic coral reef tank. The tank contains hundreds of other bony fish as well as elasmobranchs. This animal is the only representative of its species in this exhibit and was introduced directly from the wild. His medical and husbandry histories to date are unremarkable. The fish is being fed previously frozen fish and invertebrates with no vitamin supplementation. Capture of the fish and examination are made easily because the animal is resting upright on the bottom of the tank.

i. Using an appropriate sedative, what grouping of initial diagnostic tests would probably yield the most useful information in this case?
A Skin scrape, gill biopsy, blood collection for complete blood count and serum chemistries, including calcium, phosphorus, and calcitonin assay.
B Physical examination, skin scrape, gill biopsy, survey radiography, and neurological examination.
C Physical examination, skin scrape, gill biopsy, abdominal ultrasound, blood collection for complete blood count and serum chemistries, including calcium, phosphorus, and calcitonin assay.

ii. How might this animal be treated?
A Strict tank rest, feed vitamin-supplemented fish, re-radiograph in four weeks.
B Attempt surgical reduction of subluxation and maintenance with external fixator.
C There is no real hope, the animal should be killed painlessly.

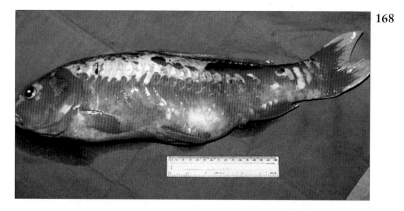

168

168 Describe the abnormality seen in the photograph (168). What are the possible differential diagnoses, and what further tests are required to make a specific diagnosis?

167 i. B. Physical examination, skin scrape, gill biopsy, survey radiography, and neurological examination.

External examination revealed a slight abrasion on the most rostral portion of the lower jaw and a relatively darkened integument over the caudal one-third of the body. Skin scrape and gill biopsy revealed no parasites but some excess mucus covering the respiratory epithelium. On neurologic examination it appeared that the animal could

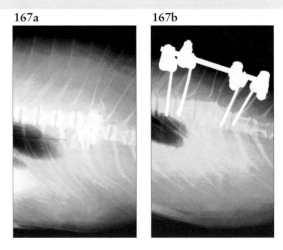

167a 167b

not sense noxious stimuli on its tail and appeared to be paralyzed in the caudal one-third of the body. Radiography revealed a spinal fracture and subluxation (**167a**). It appears that the animal made contact with some object in the tank and subsequently fractured its spine.

ii. A or B. In this case a surgical reduction was attempted with an external fixator (**167b**). A lateral approach was used and two pins were placed cranial and caudal to the lesion site. It was necessary to balance the stainless steel hardware with small amounts of closed-cell foam floatation to allow the animal to maintain an upright position. The animal began to eat and show signs of improvement; however, it was found dead about two weeks after surgery. Gross pathologic examination revealed a black cottony mass in the dorsocaudal region of the swim bladder. It has been reported that uncomplicated spinal fractures have healed with tank rest.

168 The photograph shows a koi carp with a swelling in the midline of the posterior abdomen. This had been developing over two months and the fish had gradually gone off its food and had not eaten for over a week. On palpation the mass appeared firm and the asymmetric nature of the lesion made it unlikely to be the result of free fluid or eggs within the abdominal cavity.

A needle aspirate was performed and the collected fluid failed to give any useful information on analysis. A presumptive diagnosis of neoplasia was made and euthanasia performed.

At necropsy a large cystic mass was present in the posterior abdomen involving the intestine. Histopathology showed this to be an adenocarcinoma of the bowel.

In hindsight, ultrasonographic evaluation may have been useful to show this as a fluid-filled cystic structure.

169 An established 200-L tank of fish including pearl danios, silver hatchets, rosy barbs, red-eye tetras, and tiger barbs has just begun experiencing heavy losses.
i. What is your course of action?
ii. What is your tentative diagnosis?

170 This koi pond developed a profuse bloom of algae in early summer (**170**).
i. What factors would cause this sudden algal growth?
ii. What clinical problems are associated with these water conditions?

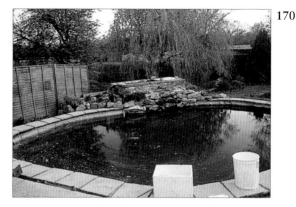

170

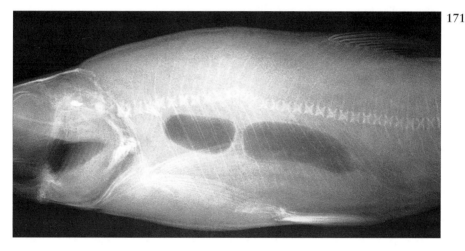

171

171 i. What feature is visible on this radiograph (**171**)?
ii. List several possible causes for this lesion.

169 i. A. Obtain a complete history. You learn that a group of blue tetras was recently added without quarantine. Two died and were removed the following day. The heater's thermostat failed and tank temperatures rose from 24°C (75.2°F) to 28°C (82.4°F) overnight. Several fish of each species listed above has died.

B. Check water quality. All parameters are acceptable except for the sudden rise in temperature.

C. Perform a physical examination. Most fish in the tank are swimming normally. One rosy barb, however, is spinning in a tight circle. One danio has bilateral exophthalmia and injected/hemorrhagic fins. No external parasites are found on skin, gills, or fins.

ii. Probably bacterial infection. You ask to sacrifice one moribund rosy barb, perform a routine necropsy, and culture the brain and kidney. While waiting for results you recommend erythromycin-medicated feed because species affected, progression, and clinical signs are very typical for streptococcal infection. It is important to realize, however, that many bacterial infections present similarly, although exophthalmia and spinning are fairly characteristic, especially in several of the species listed above. Your culture and sensitivity results will determine your drug of choice.

170 i. The growth of algae in freshwater fish ponds depends on temperature, light, and nutrient supply. Fresh nutrients are provided by the addition of tap water to top off the pond following evaporation or during routine water changes. The run off of fertilizer from the soil may add further nutrients to the pond water.

ii. Although algae produce oxygen by photosynthesis during the day, they extract oxygen from the water at night. Without extra aeration using air stones, waterfalls, fountains, or a venturi, the dissolved oxygen may drop to lethal levels and cause fish to die from anoxia, typically in the early morning hours.

Algae take up carbon dioxide from the water during daylight hours and this produces an increase in pH. The amount of increase is determined by the buffering capacity of the water and the rate of photosynthesis. In this pond an electronic meter revealed a pH of 11.0 at midday. In addition to indirect stress, the clinical effects of high pH levels include damage to the skin and gills, corneal opacity, increased toxicity of ammonia, and often death from metabolic alkalosis.

171 i. Dislocated spine between the 11th and 12th vertebrae.
ii. Inherited:

• Gene damage during egg development.

Acquired:

• Physical: trauma, electrical, tumor.
• Infection: bacterial, fungal.
• Nutritional deficiency: tryptophan, vitamin C, phosphorus.
• Chemical toxicity: pesticides, herbicides, heavy metals.

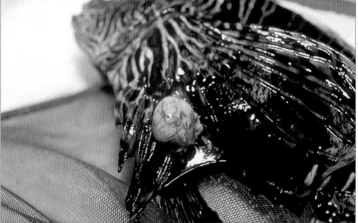

172 This lionfish presented with a large, yellow, firm round mass on the left pectoral fin near its attachment to the body (172). The fish was housed in a 88,000-L aquarium containing many lionfish. Other lionfish in the exhibit appear normal and the water quality parameters were within normal limits.
i. How would one proceed with a physical examination of this fish?
ii. What are the possible causes of the lesion observed in this fish?
iii. How would you manage this case?

173 This anemone is being buffeted by strong currents (173). Why is this so vital for the well-being of these invertebrates?

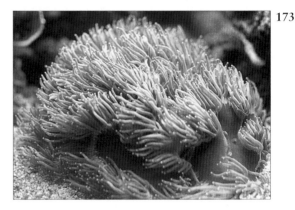

174 A local neighbor has asked your advice on how to check water quality in his ornamental pond and his fish tanks which are housed indoors.
What tests would you recommend for your neighbor to perform routinely?

172 i. Fish of the Family Scorpaenidae are venomous and should be handled with extreme care. Lionfish have a protein venom in their dorsal spines. Direct contact with this venom usually results in extreme pain at the puncture site. The venom is denatured by heat. The treatment of choice for lionfish venom is the frequent application of hot water (as hot as can be tolerated) to the puncture site. To minimize the risk of being punctured by a spine during handling, it is best to anesthetize the fish. Tricaine methanesulfonate (MS-222) is the anesthetic of choice. During handling, one should avoid contact with the dorsal spines. As a precaution, the dorsal spines should be removed before performing a necropsy.

ii. An inflammatory response, such as a granuloma, should be first on the rule-out list. Granulomas result from chronic inflammatory lesions associated with an infectious (bacterial, fungal, viral, parasitic) or chemical cause (the proteinaceous venom from another lionfish). Another possibility would be a cutaneous neoplasm.

iii. After the lionfish was properly anesthetized with MS-222 (100 p.p.m.), the mass was examined more closely. It was firm, broad-based, pedunculated, and easily excised using a scalpel blade. A small drop of cyanoacrylate glue was applied to the skin wound to form a protective seal. Cytologic examination of the tissue revealed a macrophagic inflammatory response. No etiologic agent could be found. Microbial culture was negative for bacteria and fungi. Histopathology revealed a granulomatous inflammation with no etiologic agent observed. It was presumed that the inflammatory lesion may have resulted from the sting of another lionfish.

173 Respiration in sessile invertebrates such as anemones and corals is achieved by simple diffusive gaseous exchange. In cross-section, coelenterates consist of an outer epidermal layer, an intervening mesogleal layer, and an inner gastrodermal layer. Both the epidermal and gastrodermal cells are in direct contact with water, either externally or within the coelomic cavity. In large anemones, there are often many internal, longitudinally radiating folds of the gastrodermis, called mesenteries. These mesenteries increase the internal surface area for gaseous exchange.

Tropical marine corals and anemones evolved in the surge zones, where not only is there a high pO_2 but water currents prevent a significant static zone of water developing around them. Such a zone would rapidly become depleted of oxygen as a result of the invertebrates' respiration. Due to these factors, certain invertebrates require strong currents in aquaria, stronger than is provided by standard air pumps. Power filters are preferred, and several companies now market surge systems which control multiple power heads, thereby mimicking natural current patterns.

174 The basic tests to run would be pH, temperature, total ammonia nitrogen (to calculate un-ionized ammonia), nitrite, nitrate, alkalinity, and total hardness. Although it would be helpful to know dissolved oxygen levels, the test can be difficult to perform and would soon discourage the neighbor from testing further. Tests such as alkalinity, hardness, nitrate, and nitrite are more likely to be needed when a tank or pond is first established, whereas pH, ammonia, temperature, and possibly nitrite should be tested on a regular basis. For marine systems, salinity or specific gravity testing is essential.

175 What testing regime would you recommend for the neighbor in **174**?

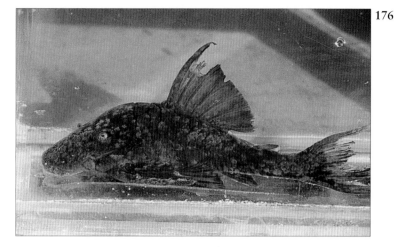

176

176 A blue-eyed plecostomus has begun to develop small, irregular, gray–white lesions on its skin (**176**). It is in a tank with several other blue-eyes. Water quality evaluation and skin, fin, and gill biopsy results are unremarkable. What are your recommendations?

177 An angelfish breeder has recently moved 20 pairs of his best breeders to a new facility. He has been unable to raise fry beyond seven to ten days of age. The breeders appear unthrifty, but none has died. Egg number and quality has markedly declined. A complete necropsy of two adult fish and six fry failed to reveal any infectious agents. Water quality analysis is unremarkable. A site visit is suggested by the owner. Upon walking into the building (a building that has not been in use for several years) the smell of hydrogen sulfide is overpowering. All windows have been sealed with plastic to maintain temperature, and there is no ventilation. Water flows in directly from a well, dug 40 years ago.
i. What is the greatest concern in the situation described?
ii. What should be done immediately?
iii. What needs to be done before fish can be reared successfully in the building?

175 Water quality should be checked at regular intervals. Although many fish keepers never check their water quality, it would be good practice to check water quality parameters approximately every two weeks. An element of organization helps to streamline the whole procedure. For example, temperature, dissolved oxygen, and pH can be recorded directly from the tank or pond as water samples are being taken. The test kits now available in many aquarium stores need only a few milliliters of water. The water should always be taken in clean glass containers kept especially for this purpose. The tests should be carried out as soon as possible after the sample has been taken. If samples must be stored, they should be kept cool in the refrigerator. All results should be recorded. It is very useful to look back at water quality records. This often helps pinpoint the start of a disease problem. It might also be possible to cooperate with neighboring aquarists so that several water samples are taken and measured at the same time. (This might even be a lucrative service for veterinary practices!)

176 A. Isolate or quarantine the sick fish and keep a close eye on the other blue-eyes in the tank. If water changes can be performed without stressing the fish, then do so.
   B. Two days later, the fish has many more raised areas on its skin and fins, with older lesions coalescing to form large areas of necrotic hemorrhagic tissue. What do you suggest now?
   C. Send fin and skin biopsy samples off for virology testing. This blue-eye is showing signs which are fairly classic in their appearance and progression for an epithelial disease most probably caused by a herpesvirus. Although rigorous isolation and experimental transmission studies have not been performed, herpesvirus-like particles have been visualized several times in skin and internal organs of affected fish. Similar lesions in other species including Pacific cod, pike, and dogfish have also been associated with herpesviruses. Usually the onset of disease in blue-eyes follows a major stress, such as shipping and poor water quality. Treatment with antiviral agents such as acyclovir have been attempted without success.

177 i. The greatest concern in the situation described is for human safety. A tightly closed room with detectable hydrogen sulfide can be dangerous to humans in the building. An individual working in this environment may become accustomed to the smell of the hydrogen sulfide, and therefore be less likely to leave the area when he or she should. Working in a sealed building, with no ventilation, is very dangerous under any circumstances.
ii. The building needs to be ventilated immediately. Doors and windows should be opened, and left open. Fans should be put in place to maximize the air movement. Fish should be removed from the building if at all possible.
iii. To solve the problem, an aeration tower needs to be constructed outside. Hydrogen sulfide is highly volatile. If the affected well water is thoroughly aerated before entering the building, the problem can be quickly, and inexpensively, resolved. A number of companies are available to do this type of work.

178 A freshwater angelfish breeder has experienced substantial loss (20%) of juvenile fish over the past two weeks. Approximately 50% of surviving fish appear lethargic, are hanging in corners of their tank, and are only picking at food that is offered. A gray film covers the dorsal surface of some of the darker varieties (i.e. black marble veil), visible when the dorsal aspect of fish are examined with indirect light. Strands of mucus are streaming from the fins of individual fish. Many animals are experiencing respiratory distress and additional mortalities are expected. A gill biopsy is pictured (×100) (**173**).

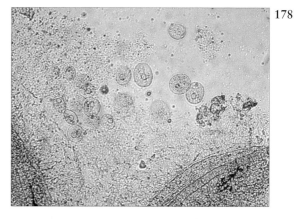

i. Which external pathogens are notorious for contributing to heavy mucus production?
ii. Which tissues should be examined to determine whether or not these are present?
iii. How serious is this problem? What steps should the owner follow to minimize losses?

179 This eight-year-old oscar presented with a three-month history of anorexia, weight loss, a buoyancy disorder, and a large inflamed mass involving the ventral abdomen (**179a**).
i. What conditions would be on your list of differentials?
ii. How would you make a noninvasive diagnosis before death?

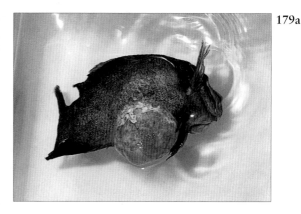

180 What are the main hematopoietic organs in a fish?

178–180: Answers

178 i. *Chilodonella* is a motile, ciliated parasite that causes external irritation and heavy mucus production. *Ichthyobodo* (Costia) is a flagellate which has also been associated with heavy mucus production on a variety of freshwater and saltwater fish. The two are readily differentiated by examining a wet mount of infected tissue at low power with a light microscope.

ii. *Chilodonella* is found on the external surfaces of fish, including gills, fins, skin, and scales. A simple scraping of affected sites is usually diagnostic (**178**).

iii. Untreated *Chilodonella* can contribute to substantial morbidity and mortality of aquarium fish. Freshwater angelfish seem to be particularly sensitive to it. Because of its direct life-cycle it is relatively easy to control. Any of the standard chemicals used to kill external parasites (salt, potassium permanganate, copper sulfate, and formalin) are effective in controlling *Chilodonella*. In recirculating systems, permanent addition of 1.0 p.p.t. salt is helpful in alleviating chronic *Chilodonella* problems.

179 i. Herniated swim bladder; herniated bowel or other abdominal viscera; neoplasia.

ii. This lateral radiograph shows a grossly enlarged radiolucent swim bladder that has herniated through the body wall (**179b**). Abdominal viscera have been forced cranially and caudally in the distended abdomen. Air was removed with a needle and syringe but the fish died despite supportive care. The etiology of this condition is unknown.

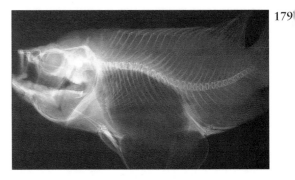

180 The main hematopoietic organs of the fish are the thymus, head kidney (**180**) (and to a much lesser extent the trunk kidney) and spleen. However, hematopoiesis can occur anywhere along the reticuloendothelial stroma of the vascular system and its associated organs.

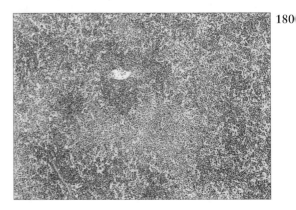

181 An adult sea raven presents with a severely distended abdomen, an elevated respiratory rate and mouth gaping. The fish was collected from the wild two years ago as an adult and placed directly into a 8,700-L tank with several other adult sea ravens and other cold marine ground fish. The animals are being maintained at a nearly constant temperature of 12.8°C (55°F). Lighting cycles are erratic. The animal's tankmates appear normal. The aquarist does not know if this animal has been eating or not and does not have any previous weights of the animals in this exhibit.

i. Using an appropriate sedative, what grouping of initial diagnostic tests would likely yield the most useful information in this case?

A Skin scrape, gill biopsy, blood collection for complete blood count and serum chemistries, including progesterone assay.

B Physical examination, skin scrape, gill biopsy, and survey radiography.

C Physical examination, skin scrape, gill biopsy, and abdominal ultrasonography.

D Physical examination, skin scrape, gill biopsy, abdominal ultrasonogaphy, blood collection for complete blood count and serum chemistries, including progesterone assay.

ii. How might this situation be treated?

A Treat the system with copper sulfate at about 0.2 p.p.m. for about three weeks; remove this animal from the system and humanely kill it so as not to re-infect the system.

B Treat the system with copper sulfate at about 0.2 p.p.m. for about three weeks; remove this animal from the system and treat it with a series of three or four formalin dips (250 p.p.m.) for ten minutes, once a week. Maintain the animal in a darkened tank.

C There is no real hope, this animal and its tankmates should be killed painlessly and the system sterilized with a hypochlorite solution.

182 A koi pond owner contacts you and complains that most of his 30 koi are scratching and flashing in his 9,500-L outdoor pond. He claims his water quality is good and mentions the fact that he added six new fish five weeks ago, which he purchased from a wholesaler. He has not lost any fish yet and adds that he thinks he can see small dark 'discs' moving across the skin of some fish. The fish pictured here has 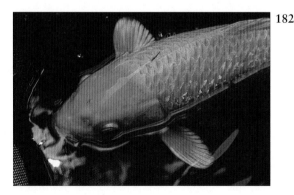 182

been caught for closer inspection (**182**). You go to the pond to investigate the problem.

i. What is at the top of your differential list?

ii. What will your diagnostic work-up consist of?

iii. Once you have the correct diagnosis, how will you treat this problem?

iv. What preventive medicine recommendations will you make?

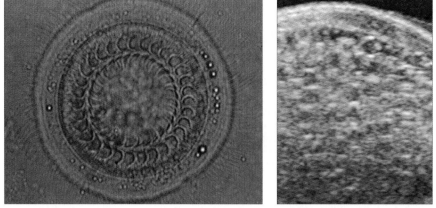

181 i. C. Physical examination revealed a severely distended abdomen that appeared to be fluid filled. The animal's gills were a hazy gray color and the gill biopsy showed that the respiratory epithelium was infested with a protozoal parasite, *Trichodina* (181a). Further examination with ultrasonography showed that the animal's abdomen was filled with roe (181b).
ii. B. If this treatment is followed, it is possible that the animal will resorb the eggs and return to normal. The fish should be monitored closely to make sure no other complications arise such as a bacterial infection of the roe. If all goes well, the animal may be returned to the exhibit tank. The long-term prognosis is unknown.

182 i. An ectoparasitic infection.
ii. The diagnostic work-up will consist of: (A) a thorough history; (B) complete water quality test; and (C) skin, fins, and gill biopsies.

iii. These fish were infected with the crustacean parasite, *Argulus*. This parasite is commonly referred to as the 'fish louse.' A parasite can be seen on the dorsal surface of the head of the fish (182). Once a pond is infected, the only way to eliminate the parasites, aside from draining the pond and removing the fish, is to treat the water with an organophosphate or a chitin synthesis inhibitor.
iv. Like most crustaceans, *Argulus* lays eggs and these hatch into a microscopic free-swimming larval form which eventually finds a fish and completes its life cycle as a skin parasite. The eggs are usually deposited on plants, rocks, or other firm submerged surfaces. Fish infected with the early life stages will look normal and the parasites will not be visible to the naked eye until they mature. The best way to prevent this condition is to quarantine all new fish for at least six weeks and monitor them closely for signs of ectoparasitic disease. If quarantine is not possible, new fish may be dipped in salt water (35 g/L) for 3–5 minutes in an effort to kill larval stages. This dip will not usually kill the adult parasites but it may force them off the fish.

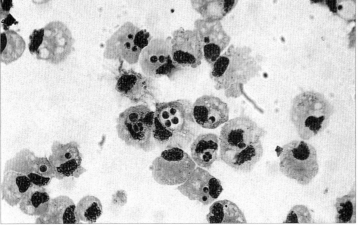

183a

183 American oysters from the Chesapeake Bay are kept in a marine tank, supplied by natural sea water, on the US mid-Atlantic coast. During their second summer, oysters begin to die.
i. How do you nonlethally obtain a hemolymph sample from an oyster?
ii. Based on the stained cytospin sample of hemocytes (**183a**), what is your diagnosis, and how would you manage the disease?

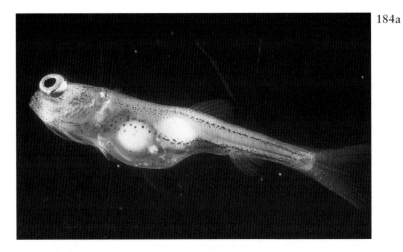

184a

184 Several large, white, focal masses are present in the viscera of this *Notho-branchius* killifish (**184a**).
What is your diagnosis?

183 **i.** Drill a hole on the flat valve near the straighter edge, located as shown, well away from the viscera, where only the mantle will be damaged by the drill entry. Direct a 3.7-cm small-gauge needle in the direction of the hinge (**183b**). The heart is located between one-third and one-half of the distance to the hinge, adjacent to the adductor muscle. Examine the clear hemolymph microscopically to ensure there is no contamination from intestinal contents or seawater. If not used for repeated hemolymph sampling, the shell defect will eventually be repaired by the mantle.

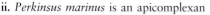

ii. *Perkinsus marinus* is an apicomplexan parasite that has devastated the commercial oyster fishery. The parasite invades cells of all tissues, causing extensive lysis. It can be recognized by tetrads of dividing trophozoites, and a large vacuole and eccentric nucleus of mature trophozoites (**183a**). Disease occurs at temperatures >20°C (68°F) and salinities >15 p.p.t. Changing to lower salinities and temperatures can slow progression of the disease, but the parasite can persist for a year or two in less-than-perfect conditions. Avoiding transplantation of infected oysters is the best method of prevention.

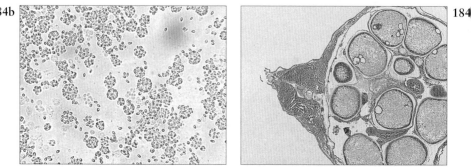

184 *Glugea*. This is a microsporidian parasite. Microsporidians are easily identified by their characteristic egg-shaped spores (**184b**). The histologic appearance of xenomas in the abdominal cavity is shown (**184c**).

185 How would you treat the problem of the fish in **184**?

186 These pictus catfish, along with numerous other species of freshwater tropical fish (tetras, cichlids, and other catfish species), died within 12 hours of being received from a local wholesaler (**186a**). The fish were truck shipped and spent six hours in their packing bags. They were allowed to acclimate to tank temperature and pH before being carefully placed in the aquaria. Over one-hundred 75-L aquaria shared a common water supply with adequate

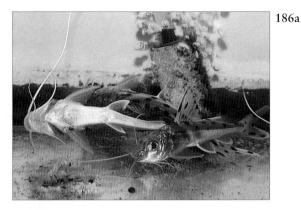
186a

aeration and biological and mechanical filtration. Standard water quality parameters were tested (ammonia, nitrite, nitrate, total alkalinity, pH, dissolved oxygen, and temperature) and all were within acceptable limits.
i. What conditions would comprise your differential list?
ii. How would you identify and correct the problem?

187 An owner complains of a recent ammonia/nitrite spike in her moderately stocked, previously healthy aquarium. One-fifth of the water is changed on a bi-weekly basis when the aquarium is healthy. Recently, multiple 50% water changes have solved the water quality problems only temporarily.

Filtration consists of an outside power filter like the one pictured here with a disposable carbon-filled filter pack (**187a**).

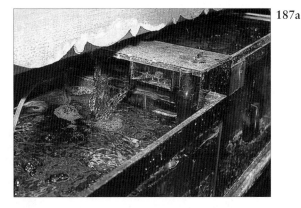
187a

Visual inspection of the filter reveals that water is passing over the top of the filter pack rather than being directed through it.
i. What is causing the alteration in water flow?
ii. How might this affect the water quality?

185 There is no proven treatment for any microsporidian parasite. A toltrazuril bath (20 p.p.m. for 1 hour every other day three times) has shown experimental efficacy against the vegetative stages, but not the spores, of *Glugea*. The best method of control is destruction of infected stocks and disinfection of facilities. This disease appears to be common in captive seahorses (**185**). Note the numerous sporocysts in this individual.

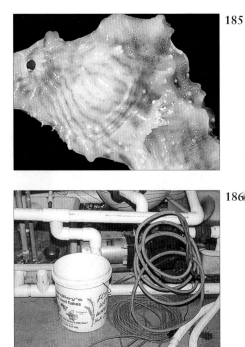

185

186 i. A toxicity of some kind is almost surely the cause of this problem. It would be extremely unlikely that a pathogen could act this quickly against such a broad range of species. The history helps to rule out any water quality shock and standard water quality values are normal. Potential toxins would include copper, other heavy metals, pesticides, and chemotherapeutics. Supersaturation (gas-bubble disease) could cause this but the fish displayed no clinical signs of this disease.

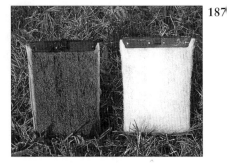

186

ii. When the water was tested for copper, levels were found to be 0.8 p.p.m. This level is very high and certainly toxic for freshwater fish, especially in soft, acidic water. After questioning several pet store employees it was discovered that several weeks before, 6 m of fresh copper tubing was installed in the sump as a heating coil to warm the water (**186b**). The copper in the system had been leaching into the water from the tubing. The tubing was removed, water changes were initiated, and a copper chelating agent was added to the system.

187 i. The alteration in water flow is most likely caused by the accumulation of particulate matter in the filter pack (**187b**) such that the flow of water through the filter is impeded. Regular rinsing and/or changing of the filter pack can prevent this from happening.
ii. When water is allowed to circumvent the filter pack, it bypasses the richest source of nitrogen-fixing bacteria, dramatically decreasing the filter's efficiency. In addition, organic compounds trapped within the filter can release toxins into the water as they break down, compounding water problems.

187

188 Why are these bags of barley straw used in outdoor fish ponds (188)?

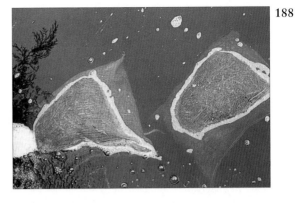

189 This koi presented with a 10-mm swelling on its caudal fin which had been noticed for a week (189).
i. What is the cause of this swelling?
ii. Suggest a course of action to treat this fish.

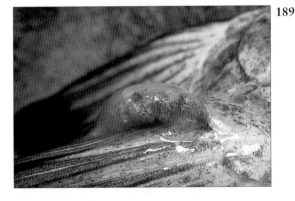

190 A mini-reef aquarium contained a wide variety of invertebrates and some smaller fish: percula clownfish, wreckfish, and damselfish. Over several months there has been a gradual decline in several of the sessile invertebrates, including the soft corals (190). Lighting appeared fine – indeed, both algae and tridachnid clams were thriving. What would be your next step to investigate this problem?

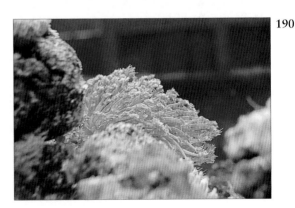

188 When barley straw decomposes aerobically in freshwater it produces various chemicals that inhibit the growth of algae. These chemicals are produced after the straw has been soaking for about a month and continues for six months. Experiments have shown that 5 g of straw per 1,000 L is required with a minimum of 100 g being used. The anti-algal factors are only generated when the straw is decomposing in water containing sufficient dissolved oxygen and exposure to sunlight. Good movement of water through the straw with monthly inspection and agitation is recommended. This method of control is more effective on unicellular algae than filamentous blanketweed. However, it should be noted that anaerobic decomposition of straw produces a foul, rotting smell and the release of toxic breakdown products which may affect fish health.

189 i. This swelling is due to *Dermocystidium koi*, an unusual fungal-like infection. The characteristic white hyphae visible under the skin release thousands of spores into the water. These spores can be identified by microscopic examination of a wet preparation of hyphae plucked from the lesion. Spores contain a large central vacuole or refractile body with the cytoplasm and nucleus restricted to the narrow periphery; spores are up to 15 μm in diameter, about the size of an erythrocyte.
ii. Surgical removal of the lesions prior to rupture and topical dressing of the wound to avoid secondary bacterial infection is recommended. It is not yet known if this disease infects other fish species, and although usually only a few koi are affected, environmental treatment with an antifungal product may be warranted.

190 Basic water quality parameters need to be checked. The results were:

Temperature: 26°C (78.8°F)
pH: 8.1
Ammonia: negative
Nitrite: negative
Nitrate: 100 p.p.m.
Hardness: 286 p.p.m. as $CaCO_3$
Specific gravity: 1.022
Redox potential: 25 mV

All of the above parameters are acceptable apart from the nitrate levels. A level of 100 p.p.m. is far too high. For normal marine aquaria, a maximum of 40 p.p.m. is recommended, whereas for invertebrates a better level would be no more than 15 p.p.m. Some invertebrates, especially the Goniopora corals, are sensitive to nitrate and may suffer at levels greater than 20 p.p.m. Possible causes include infrequent water changes, overfeeding, or overstocking (especially with fish).

In the former case, regular partial water changes should help; reduction of stocking levels plus the addition of a denitrator should bring the nitrate levels back to the desired range. If the tapwater has high ambient nitrate levels, then use of a reverse osmosis unit to remove the nitrate before mixing new salt solutions would be in order.

191 A home aquarist recently set up a 38-L tank stocked with ten black mollies. The fish were fine for the first two weeks; however, four were found dead yesterday, and the surviving fish all appear lethargic. Two survivors have obvious unilateral exophthalmia (popeye) and one has unilateral swelling along the lateral body wall. Water quality parameters are shown below:

Dissolved oxygen: 7.4 p.p.m.
Total ammonia: 0 p.p.m.
Temperature: 24°C (75.2°F)
Nitrite: 0 p.p.m.
pH: 7.6
Salinity: 2 p.p.t.
Total alkalinity: 137 p.p.m.
Total hardness: 171 p.p.m.

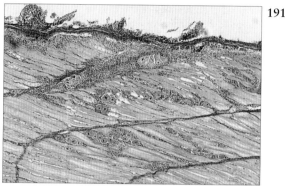
191

A wet mount of material from an affected eye revealed large numbers of the ciliated protozoan, Tetrahymena. This histologic section shows organisms within muscle (191).

i. What is the clinical significance of Tetrahymena in the described case presentation?
ii. What is the best management strategy for this problem?

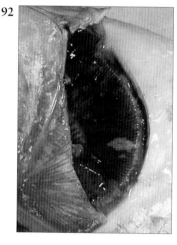
92

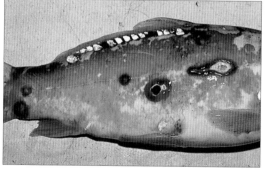
193

193 i. Describe the gross lesions (193).
ii. What are the main differentials?
iii. What further tests can be done to confirm the diagnosis?

192 i. How does the gross appearance of this gill (192) differ from normal?
ii. What is the likely cause?
iii. What is the likely sequela?

191 i. Although *Tetrahymena* may be of questionable significance when present on the external surface of fish, particularly in an organically rich environment, it is highly significant any time it is present internally. When systemic infections occur, the parasite has a great predilection for the eye and for skeletal muscle. It occasionally may be found in brain or kidney. Because of its predilection for live-bearing species, *Teterahymena* is sometimes referred to as 'guppy killer' or 'guppy disease', although it can be found in a variety of freshwater fish.

ii. When *Tetrahymena* is restricted to the external surface of fish, it is susceptible to all chemicals used to control external protozoan infestations (i.e. formalin, copper sulfate, potassium permanganate, and salt). When the parasite invades systemically, it is refractory to treatment. In the situation presented here, depopulation of the aquarium is recommended. The tank should be thoroughly disinfected before restocking.

192 i. When normal gills are examined they appear reddish-pink and the separate primary lamellae are clearly visible. In this photograph, the gills are very dark and mottled with discrete necrotic centres. This is the characteristic appearance of 'bacterial gill disease.'

ii. This condition is likely to follow any irritation of the gill resulting in gill hyperplasia. The irritation may be caused by parasites, suspended solids, toxins, or metabolic by-products.

iii. Normal gill function includes oxygen uptake, excretion of ammonia and bicarbonate, and fluid and electrolyte balance. Extensive gill necrosis can be debilitating or even fatal. In addition, bacterial colonization of the gill may lead to generalized septicemia resulting in ulceration and death.

This sequence of events occurs when fish are chronically exposed to water quality conditions that are less than adequate.

193 i. The gross appearance of the skin of this koi reveals a number of discrete lesions showing an inflamed, hyperemic, raised rim with a central necrotic core.

ii. The main differentials include an ulcerated tumor or granuloma, hypersensitivity reaction, and localized bacterial infection.

iii. Clinically, the gross appearance is different from the typical bacterial ulcer in which the lesion appears as a crater with no raised rim. Routine skin scrapings failed to reveal the presence of any parasites, and bacterial cultures failed to isolate any significant organisms.

Under benzocaine anesthesia a biopsy was taken and submitted for histopathology. The examination failed to indicate the presence of malignant cells, but showed cells typical of a hypersensitivity reaction. It was considered that the most probable cause was a severe reaction to the anchor sites of the anchor worm *Lernaea*, a crustacean ectoparasite.

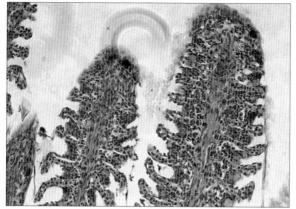

194

194 i. Describe the pathologic process occurring in the gill shown (194)?
ii. How would this disease process progress?
iii. What are the possible causes?

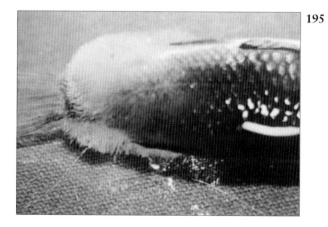

195

195 i. Identify the organism in the photograph (195).
ii. How does the organism produce disease?
iii. What other factors may have been associated with the problem?

196 What are the signs of poor water quality in marine aquaria with respect to the tank conditions and the fish themselves?

194 i. The photograph shows a moderate degree of epithelial hyperplasia of the gill. The secondary lamellae have become rounded up and shortened. At the tips of the primary lamellae, the adjacent secondary lamellae have become fused.
ii. If gill irritation persists, the fusion of the secondary lamellae will continue, such that the clubbing of the whole length of the primary lamellae becomes complete. Further changes result in fusion of adjacent primary lamellae, thus obliterating any resemblance of normal gill structure.

These changes predispose to the colonization by bacteria, which cause further gill damage and necrosis. This may lead to a generalized septicemia.
iii. These changes are the result of any irritation, including external parasites, suspended solids, heavy metals, or metabolic toxins (e.g. ammonia or nitrite). The reduced blood supply to the tissue increases the susceptibility to bacterial invasion. The common names for this condition are 'environmental gill disease' and 'bacterial gill disease.'

195 i. The photograph shows the fine cotton-like appearance typical of infection with the water mold *Saprolegnia*. Such lesions are more easily visualized when the fish is in the water. The examination of a wet preparation under the microscope will indicate the presence of the characteristic branched aseptate hyphae.
ii. The zoospores of the fungus attach to damaged skin where they germinate to produce hyphae. Proteolytic enzymes are then secreted that damage surrounding tissue, thus encouraging the spread of the lesion.
iii. In general, this is considered a secondary, opportunistic infection. In most cases the fish need to be weakened by stresses such as parasitic infestation or poor management leading to water quality problems. Compromise of the integrity of the integument is a predisposing factor. Once an infection becomes established in a pond or aquarium, the concentration of zoospores in the water may rise to such a level that even otherwise healthy fish succumb.

196 Frothiness, cloudiness, and malodor are signs of poor water quality. If it is obvious that evaporative losses have occurred and the aquarium has not been topped up with fresh water, you should conclude that regular water quality checks have not been performed. Overgrowth of algae on stones, gravel, and the walls of the aquarium indicate that there might be too much light, not enough manual cleaning of the aquarium, or both.

The fish may lose their colorful appearance, they may have frayed fins, abnormal swimming posture, and occasionally they may show rapid opercular movements indicating difficulty in extracting oxygen from the water. This environment then becomes suitable for secondary parasitic infestation and very soon the whole tank of fish is sick. In time, fungal or bacterial infections may affect the fish. It is equally possible for fish to succumb to a parasitic infection, which then predisposes them to secondary bacterial or fungal disease.

197 A sunset thick-lipped gourami weighing 8 g is examined because of a 5 mm diameter midventral abdominal mass. A fine-needle aspirate reveals only red blood cells and thrombocytes. A barium gastrointestinal study is performed to help determine visceral involvement in the swelling (197a).

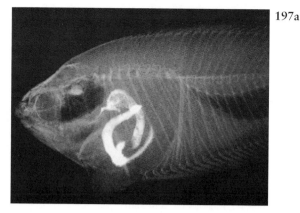

i. Identify the two radiolucent areas.

ii. List some differential diagnoses for the abdominal mass.

198 A client contacts you and is concerned that her silver dollars are sick. She recently purchased them from a pet store and placed the five fish in her 200-L community aquarium. Like the fish pictured here, all five had distinct, raised, black spots on their skin that looked like poppy seeds (198). The fish were be-

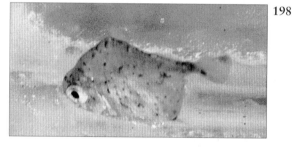

having normally and the rest of the fish in the tank were fine. The owner did not notice the spots in the pet store but remembers seeing them shortly after introducing the fish to her well-lit aquarium.

i. What are these spots?

ii. What is the life cycle of this parasite?

iii. Why are the nodules black?

iv. Can or should this condition be treated?

199 This orfe had been owned for a year and was kept in a garden pond. It had difficulty swimming for the past five months and was getting progressively worse (199).

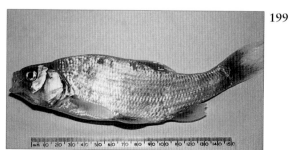

i. Describe the abnormal posture of this fish.

ii. Suggest a method of investigation.

197 i. The cranial radiolucent area is the labyrinth organ. Fish of the Family Anabantidae use this organ to extract atmospheric oxygen, supplementing oxygen absorbed by the gills. The caudal radiolucent area is the swim bladder.

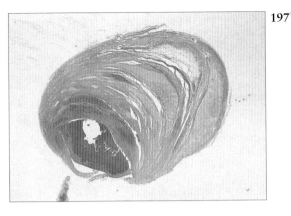

ii. Differentials include neoplasia (e.g. carcinoma of epithelial origin, fibrosarcoma, hepatic tumor), abscess, hernia (without intestinal involvement), parasitic cyst, and hematoma. On excisional biopsy the mass had a sessile base communicating with the coelomic cavity. Histologic diagnosis (entire mass in histologic cross-section shown) was a consolidated hematoma of undetermined origin (**197b**). The mass did not recur.

198 i. These spots represent the encysted metacercaria of a digenetic trematode, most likely belonging to the genus *Neascus*. This condition is common in wild-caught silver dollars and related characins.

ii. The fish is an intermediate host for this parasite. The definitive host is usually a fish-eating bird; a molluscan invertebrate, usually a snail, is the first intermediate host.

iii. In most cases the black color of the cysts is caused by a host reaction to the parasite and melanin is deposited around the encysted metacercaria.

iv. This condition is not harmful to the fish and cannot be transmitted to other fish in the aquarium without the definitive and first intermediate hosts being present. Many pet store clerks call this condition 'salt and pepper' and will commonly advise customers that the condition is not harmful to the fish. There is evidence that treatment using parasiticides that target trematodes (praziquantel, 5–10 p.p.m. for 24 hours as a bath immersion) will kill the metacercaria; however, the pigmented cysts will likely remain for some time.

199 i. Lordosis.

ii. Radiography will demonstrate the extent of any spinal deformity.

200 Your hospital provides veterinary care for a small chain of pet stores. Most of your interaction has been focused on the mammals and birds in the shops, but the owners have asked you to help them with a continuing problem of mortalities in their tropical fish. Newly arrived fish look fine, but after a few days, they break with various diseases and die. This has been happening for a long time, but the scale of the losses has received the attention of the owner. The problem occurs in each of the five stores and the problem is sporadic with regard to which species of fish are affected.
  How would you assist your client?

201 This anesthetized tilapia is being bled from the caudal vein located directly ventral to the vertebral column (**201a**). The picture illustrates a lateral approach to the vessel.
i. What is another commonly used approach?
ii. Why is the use of glass syringes discouraged in fish?
iii. How should the plastic syringes be treated before use?

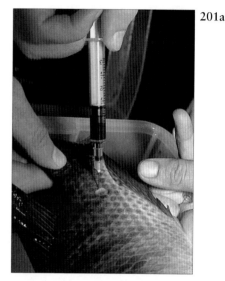

201a

202 A tropical marine aquarium has been in operation for a long period of time (**202**). Water quality checks are not carried out as frequently as they should be. It is apparent that the pH is slowly failing. The fish appear healthy. Some new fish which have very specific water quality requirements are introduced and within days they die. What is the relevance of the declining pH, and what should you do to correct the situation?

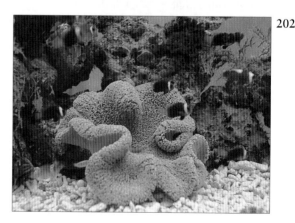

202

200 Visits to each of the stores to examine the fish holding systems and ideally the process of unpacking and adding new fish are warranted and will help you identify potential problems caused by procedures in the stores. If shipping and mortality records are available, they should be carefully examined for patterns. Otherwise, you should urge the owner to institute a careful record system to help identify whether specific wholesalers might be responsible for the affected fish.

It is common for retail stores to mix new arrivals with unsold fish and to hold them in very high density. Sales display tanks are often on large multi-tank systems sharing the water among a wide variety of species. Rarely are multiple tanks available for a single species of fish and certain species such as the armored catfish are frequently spread out with a few in each tank. If records do not point to specific sources of problem fish and inspections of the stores do not identify husbandry methods likely to be responsible for the problems, you should ask the owner to consider instituting a truncated quarantine regimen. Although most pet fish retailers cannot afford a full quarantine, it is sometimes possible to identify a set of tanks that can be used to hold new arrivals for a week or longer. With most outbreaks occurring shortly after shipping trauma, and combined with strategically grouping incoming shipments, even this short isolation can be very beneficial. It may also be possible to modify the water in the quarantine tanks by adding low levels of salt to control protozoans and reduce nitrite stresses.

201 i. The ventral approach is often productive in fish with a thick caudal peduncle like this clown triggerfish (**201b**).
ii. In general, fish blood coagulates very quickly and contact with glass facilitates this clotting.
iii. It is best to coat plastic syringes with lithium heparin before phlebotomy is performed. This can be accomplished by drawing the heparin solution from the bottle, filling the syringe, and then injecting the heparin back into the bottle.

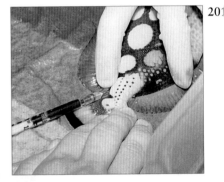

201

202 A decline in pH in a marine aquarium indicates that the sea water is ageing and its buffering capacity is declining. The situation might be acceptable for fish already living in the tank but a newly introduced fish may succumb to the poor water quality. The best recourse is to carry out a series of partial (up to 25%) water changes. It is worth thinking about species tolerance at this time. Although it is tempting to give a general value that is good for any particular water quality parameter, this is very dangerous, e.g. up to 40 p.p.m. nitrate should be acceptable to fish, although some invertebrates can only tolerate up to 5 p.p.m. The golden rule should always be that optimal environmental conditions should be checked for every living thing in a tank. Do not use metal implements in marine aquaria because toxic ions can leach into the water.

203 Piscivorous birds such as herons (203a) and cormorants can be serious predators of ornamental pond fish causing loss, damage, and stress. What measures can be taken to reduce the risk of bird predation?

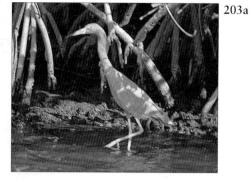

203a

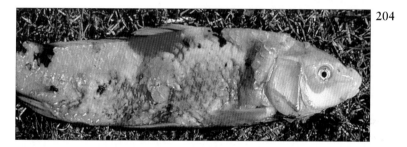

204

204 The photograph of this koi carp shows gross emaciation (204).
i. What are the probable differential diagnoses?
ii. What further tests can be done to make a specific diagnosis?

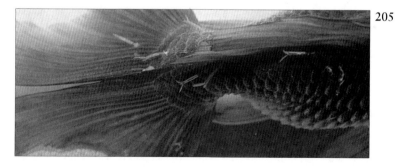

205

205 Several Y-shaped parasites are found attached to the skin of a black Moor goldfish (205).
i. What species of parasite is this?
ii. What treatment is recommended?

203 Ensure that the pond is deep enough and provide plants and structures within the pond to allow the fish to seek refuge. Ensure that pond sides are steep enough not to allow birds to land and stand at the pond edges. Wires or monofilament line over the pond can be used to prevent access but these must be high enough not to allow birds to use the wires as perches to obtain fish. Monofilament

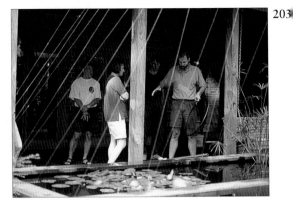

fishing line has been used for this purpose around this koi pond (**203b**). Artificial predatory birds and other decoys may act as deterrents.

204 **i.** The photograph shows severe emaciation that had developed over three to four months. The probable differential diagnoses are: chronic parasitism; chronic granulomatous disease; neoplasia.

ii. Palpation revealed almost a complete lack of normal body musculature with protrusion of the underlying bony prominences. No abdominal mass could be palpated. The prognosis was considered to be hopeless and the fish was killed painlessly.

At necropsy, multiple grayish granulomas were present in the viscera. The examination of impression smears indicated the presence of acid-fast staining organisms. Histopathology confirmed the presence of granulomas with necrotic centers typical of those seen in infections with mycobacteria.

Mycobacterium fortuitum is the most frequently isolated species in fresh or brackish water fish, whereas *Mycobacterium marinum* is seen in marine fish. The infection is usually transmitted orally, but can occur through wounds or by way of external parasites. Overcrowding is a common predisposing factor and hence imported farmed fish are always a potential source of infection. The long incubation period (at least six weeks) adds to the practical difficulty of identifying infected fish at the time of import.

205 **i.** Anchorworm, *Lernaea cyprinacea*.

ii. Control of this parasite requires manual removal of these egg-laying adult stages, preferably under sedation or general anesthesia. The anchoring points on the fish's skin should be treated topically to avoid secondary bacterial or fungal infection and ulceration. Environmental control of the immature parasites will require the use of an organophosphate or a chitin synthesis inhibitor. The use of these products may be restricted in some areas.

206 The figure shows the normal microscopic structure of a gill (206).
i. What are the functions of the gill?
ii. How does the anatomic structure aid these functions?
iii. How does hyperplasia affect the structure and function of the gills?

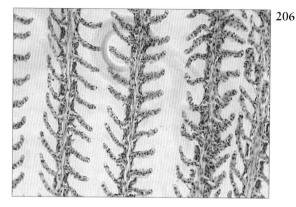

206

207 This electric eel has been maintained uneventfully in a 1,100-L display tank for the past six months (207a). It suddenly developed a dramatic swelling behind the head. You anesthetize the eel and take the radiograph shown (207b).
i. What is your radiographic diagnosis?
ii. What is your further diagnostic plan?

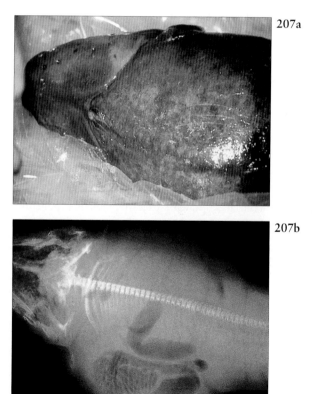

207a

207b

206 i. The functions of the gill are:

- Respiration. The gill is the site of gas exchange, where dissolved oxygen in the aquatic environment diffuses into the blood, and carbon dioxide diffuses out.
- Nitrogenous excretion. Unlike mammals, where nitrogenous waste is excreted in the form of urea in the urine, this route accounts for only about 10% of nitrogenous waste excretion in fish. The majority is excreted through the gill in the form of ammonia. Ammonia is very soluble in water, forming ammonium and hydroxyl ions. The ammonia and ammonium ions are then either washed away or metabolized by bacteria to nitrite and then nitrate as part of the nitrogen cycle.
- Fluid balance. To maintain the correct fluid balance, there are active transport mechanisms in the gill to regulate sodium and chloride concentrations. In freshwater fish, this involves the uptake of sodium ions (in exchange for ammonium and hydrogen ions) and chloride ions (in exchange for bicarbonate ions). In marine fish, the problem is reversed and sodium and chloride ions are actively excreted.

ii. To perform these functions, the blood and the water must be separated by only a very thin layer of tissue. The gill surface available for exchange must also be as large as possible. This is achieved by the anatomic arrangement of the gill filaments which are divided into multiple finger-like processes, the primary lamellae, which in turn are subdivided into secondary lamellae. The membrane covering the secondary lamellae provides the exchange surface. Under normal circumstances there is very little mucus produced at the gill lamellar surfaces.

Gill function is additionally facilitated by the continuous passage of water over the gill surface resulting from the unidirectional pumping action of the buccal cavity and opercula.

iii. Hyperplasia results in shortening and rounding of the secondary lamellae. As the condition progresses, adjacent secondary lamellae fuse resulting in clubbing. This greatly reduces the surface area available for exchange. The irritants causing hyperplasia also stimulate excessive mucus production, which further compromises gill function.

207 i. This fish shows dramatic abdominal distension caused by accumulation of coelomic fluid, compatible with a diagnosis of ascites.

ii. A coeliocentesis was performed, removing several milliliters of a clear sterile transudate. The coelom refilled with fluid within 24 hours. Evaluation of the water quality of the tank was unremarkable with the exception of a pH of 7.8. The normal habitat of this fish is in mud streams and pools of northern South America and Central America where pH is routinely below 6.0. A diagnosis of chronic alkalosis, resulting in inability to compensate for water balance through the exchange of hydrogen ions at the gill, was made. Adjusting the pH to 6.5 resulted in rapid resolution of the ascites, which did not recur.

208 Several fish in a marine community tank are scratching, 'flashing', and exhibiting rapid respiration. No external irregularities are seen on the integument.
What should you do?

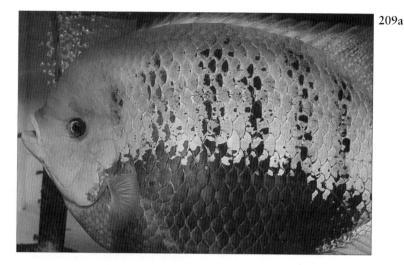

209a

209 This 2-kg Pearci cichlid presented with a three-week history of anorexia and failure to produce feces (209a). The fish broke a submersible aquarium heater one month ago. Gastrointestinal obstruction is high on your differential list.
i. What diagnostic technique will you use to rule out gastrointestinal obstruction?
ii. How will you apply this technique?

210 This 11-year-old comet goldfish lives alone in a 75-L aquarium with undergravel filtration (210). The fish presented with anorexia of a week's duration and areas of petechiation at the base of the dorsal fin and along the back. While taking the history, you learn that the owner rarely changes water (only replaces water lost due to evaporation). The fish has lived alone for five years and is fed flake food and some pellets.
What is your diagnostic plan for this case and how will you manage the problem?

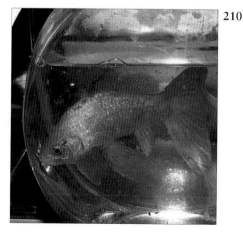

210

208 One of the fish exhibiting these signs should be captured and removed from the tank. Perform a skin scrape on the fish. The sample is placed on a clean microscope slide and a simple wet mount is prepared, using water from the tank. If the fish had been exhibiting respiratory distress, a gill biopsy can also be performed by gently lifting the operculum and snipping several gill lamellae. Protozoan parasites are the most common cause of the type of irritation and distress described in the question. If protozoans are present, they will be easily recognized, and will probably be active. Ciliates such as *Cryptocaryon* or dinoflagellates such as *Amyloodinium* can usually be identified. If no ectoparasites are found, the fish should be returned to the tank and the occupants observed very closely for the next several days. A re-examination is recommended, especially if clinical signs persist.

209 i. Contrast radiography.
ii. After tranquilizing the fish with 150 p.p.m. tricaine methanesulfonate, a flexible rubber catheter is used to introduce 5 ml/kg (10 ml) of iohexol 300 into the stomach. Iohexol is a low osmolar, non-ionic water soluble contrast media that is safe when administered intravenously, intrathecally, or orally. Serial radiographs are then made until the contrast media is excreted. The radiographs pictured were made at time zero (**209b**) and 10 minutes (**209c**). Note that after 10 minutes the iohexol has already filled the stomach, proximal intestine, and a small amount can be seen in the lower intestine. This fish did not have an impaction, but it took nearly five days for the contrast to clear the gastrointestinal (GI) tract. Times for contrast clearance vary widely between species. Iohexol was selected due to a demonstrated decrease in transit time in

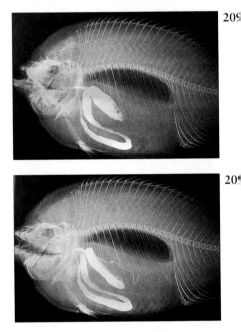

other species (bird, dog, and cat). Factors such as gut motility, length of GI tract, and metabolic rate can all affect contrast clearance.

210 After testing the water you find that the pH is 4.0 and the total ammonia nitrogen is 2.0 p.p.m. Although the ammonia is not toxic at this pH, the extremely low pH of the water is certainly a stress to the fish. Gradual water changes are in order. The owner of this fish was instructed to change 10% of the water every day for 10–14 days until the pH returned to between 7.0 and 7.5. The fish improved dramatically after the first several days and the owner was instructed to continue regular water changes at a rate of 30% per month.

211 You are called to respond to an emergency at the large outdoor shark exhibit in your aquatic park. Three sharks are floating dead and two others are thrashing at the surface as if in convulsions. It is early in the morning and the aquarists have just arrived at the exhibit to find the scene you are looking at. The exhibit is a large (nearly 1 hectare) pond dug in the coral rock of the small island where your park is located. There are six large sharks in the exhibit: one tiger shark, three large bull sharks, and two large mako sharks. The tiger shark was recently caught and has not been doing well. The others are feeding and have been in the exhibit at least five months.

The exhibit is uniformly 3.5 m deep and receives filtered sea water pumped from 1.5 km off shore. Approximately 25% of the water is changed each 24 hours. Luckily, it is raining and has been all night. You will not have to deal with large crowds when the park opens in just an hour. While you are standing on a small path overlooking the pond, you notice that the grass near the tracks of the railroad ride that runs past the exhibit is brown and dying. You ask the curator about it and he tells you that they spray the tracks every few weeks to keep the grass from derailing the train.

i. What is your highest differential?
ii. How do you proceed?

212 A koi pond has been set up for approximately two years and no new fish have been brought in since it was initially stocked. Recently, the owner has been improving the aquascape by adding beautiful, flowering water lilies. On Monday morning, following a weekend of planting new lilies in the pond, the fish are observed to be huddling near the bottom of the pond, refuse all food offered, and have an increased respiratory rate. Water quality parameters at 10.00 a.m. were:

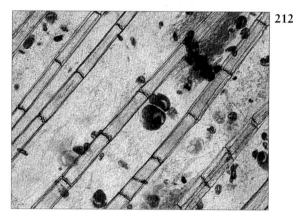
212

Dissolved oxygen: 7 p.p.m.
Total ammonia nitrogen: 1 p.p.m.
Temperature: 28°C (82.4°F)
pH: 7.2

Total alkalinity: 120 p.p.m.
Nitrite: 0 p.p.m.
Total hardness: 120 p.p.m.

Gill and fin biopsis (**212**) of an affected fish reveal numerous, motile-ciliated organisms, some with a visible horseshoe-shaped macronucleus.
i. What is causing the fish to act lethargic and depressed?
ii. What is the likely source of infection?
iii. How would you prevent this problem in the future?
iv. How should the current problem be handled?

211 i. The rapid onset of this problem, affecting several species of reasonably acclimated animals, makes toxicity a primary differential. You should be particularly concerned because of the potential for sprayed herbicides to have been washed into the exhibit by the rain.

ii. Although organophosphates or chlorinated hydrocarbons came quickly to mind because of the convulsive activities of the surviving sharks, the sprayed compound contained arsenic. Although efforts were made to change as much water as possible, all of the sharks died. The sixth shark was wedged under the inflow pipes and was dead. Postmortem examination of the sharks and subsequent analysis of liver and kidney tissues confirmed arsenic intoxication as a probable cause of death. Protocols were implemented to have all xenobiotic compounds used in the park and the procedures for their use evaluated by the veterinary staff for potential hazards to exhibit animals.

212 i. The clinical signs are suggestive of parasitic disease, although the potential for systemic illness should be recognized. In the narrative, a large, motile, ciliate with a horseshoe-shaped macronucleus was observed on the gills and fins of affected fish. The organism observed on the gill biopsy is *Ichthyophthirius multifiliis*. At water temperatures of 28°C (82.4°F), this parasite is capable of rapid replication and could cause serious disease within three to four days of introduction.

ii. A probable source for the apparent recent introduction of *I. multifiliis* to the fish population is the newly purchased lilies. Plants, nets, and other objects can serve as fomites for the encysted stage of the parasite.

iii. Plants can be quarantined for *I. multifiliis* by placing them in an aquarium which is not stocked with fish and maintaining the water temperature at 28°C (82.4°F) for at least seven days. As individual cysts rupture, emerging tomites will not have access to a new host and therefore will not survive. Careful disinfection of inanimate objects such as nets (i.e. 10 p.p.m. chlorine bleach for one hour followed by a thorough rinse) is important to avoid introduction of infectious agents during cleaning or movement of animals.

iv. To solve the immediate problem, either plants or fish should be removed from the pond as chemical treatment may damage delicate lilies. Parasite control can be achieved using a number of chemical products. Formalin would be the treatment of choice in this case, as long as adequate aeration was available. Formalin is readily available through pet stores. A concentration of 25 p.p.m. can be applied to the pond every other day for at least three treatments or until the problem is resolved.

213 A very valuable showa koi has a swollen abdomen that the owner says has increased in size over the past several months. You have performed a standard clinical work-up including fine-needle aspirate, radiographs, and ultrasonographic examination and believe the swelling to be the result of a large abdominal mass.

What sophisticated diagnostic test can be used further to characterize the size, shape, and location of the tumor?

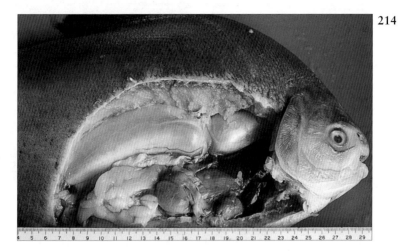

214

214 i. Identify the large bisaculate white structure in this pacu necropsy specimen (**214**).
ii. What can you say about the function, derivation, location, and histology of this organ?

215 A pregnant yellow stingray is several weeks past its expected parturition date.
What diagnostic tests would you perform to determine the status of the ray pups?

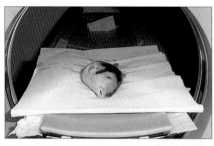

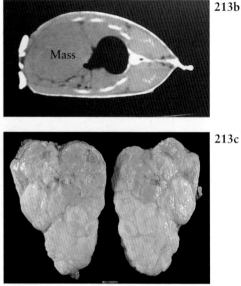

213 Computed tomography (CT). In this case the fish was anesthetized with MS-222 at a concentration of 200 p.p.m. The fish was placed in the scanner in left lateral recumbency (213a) and a series of images were obtained. The image clearly shows the large mass just ventral to the swim bladder with most of the viscera displaced to the left (213b). Surgery was performed and a 215 g sarcoma was successfully removed (213c). This fish was still doing well ten months post-operatively.

214 i. This is the swim bladder.
ii. The retroperitoneal swim bladder develops as an outpocketing of the gastrointestinal tract in most fish species. The swim bladder usually is used in buoyancy control, but in some species may function in respiration, sound production, and possibly the detection of pressure changes. The microscopic anatomy varies widely among species. Histologically, the swim bladder may closely resemble the digestive tract, or it may be reduced to a simple inner mucous membrane and thin outer layer of connective tissue. A supportive layer of smooth muscle is usually present and this layer may also contain elastic fibers. Physoclistous swim bladders contain one or more highly vascular retia mirabilia. The number and location of these retia varies between taxonomic groups. It should be noted that not all fish have swim bladders.

215 Some ray species easily conceive in captivity but dystocias are common. Visual examination and palpation of the distended coelomic wall usually indicates the health status of the ray pup(s). Healthy mature pups are generally lively and can be observed swimming inside the uterus by closely examining the body wall of the mother for their characteristic fluttering swimming motion. As the fetuses mature past term, they can die in the uterus where they are either absorbed or mummified. If fetal movement is not seen, palpation of the mother can stimulate the pups to move or ultrasonographic examination can be performed to search for fetal heartbeats. The mother may become sick if the fetuses putrefy.

216 With regard to the pregnant yellow stingray in 215, how would you resolve this dystocia?

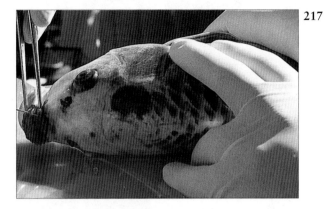

217

217 Why would you wear gloves when handling a fish (217)?

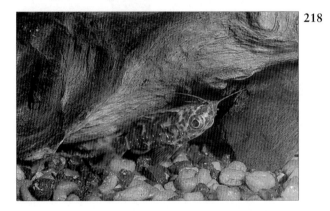

218

218 This catfish spends most of its time swimming upside down at the water's surface (218). Visitors in the waiting room of the office where the aquarium is situated comment that there is a sick fish in the tank. What is the explanation?

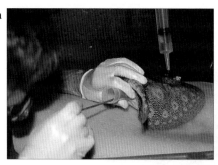

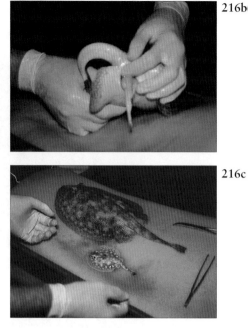

216 If the fetus(es) are alive and the known parturition date is past, the female can be anesthetized, placed on a soft moist substrate, and the cloaca examined (**216a**). In this case a smooth syringe case was used as a speculum, allowing access to the 'cervix.' A small blunt catheter can be introduced into the cervix which is dilated by rotating the catheter in a slowly expanding circular motion. Clear to cloudy uterine fluid evacuates once the cervix is expanded and a gloved finger can be introduced to continue dilating the cervix. Once the cervix is adequately dilated, the tail of the pup can be exteriorized and gentle but steady pressure is placed on the mother's body wall, expelling the pup (**216b**). If the pup cannot be extricated in this manner, the fetus can be removed by placing careful but steady traction on the venomous spine using a pair of forceps or hemostats. If the cervical dilatation is unsuccessful, the pups can be removed surgically. Yellow ray pups are miniatures of the adults (**216c**). This particular ray produced four healthy young.

217 Fish should only be handled when absolutely necessary. Handling time should always be minimized. Make sure all work done with the animal is carefully planned and thought out. If one has never worked with a particular species of fish, it is very important to learn as much as possible about that species before handling the animal. Potentially dangerous animals should never be handled alone. Fish can carry zoonotic organisms such as mycobacteria, so latex or plastic gloves should be worn when handling fish. Moistened latex gloves also protect the fish by decreasing the disruption of the protective mucus layer, which is important in osmoregulation and immune function. Eye protection will protect the fish handler from splashing water.

218 This is an upside-down catfish belonging to the genus *Synodontis*. Many species belonging to this genus and related genera utilize this swimming pattern to obtain food floating at the surface. The condition is normal.

219 A group of five medium-sized discus are housed in a 280-L circular tank. The fish have recently darkened in color, some appearing gray along the dorsal body wall. The respiratory rate is increased and the fish are not eating very well. Water quality parameters are shown below:

Dissolved oxygen: 7.8 p.p.m.
Total ammonia: 0 p.p.m.
Temperature: 29°C (84.2°F)
Nitrite: 0 p.p.m.
Total alkalinity: 51 p.p.m.
pH: 6.8
Total hardness: 51 p.p.m.

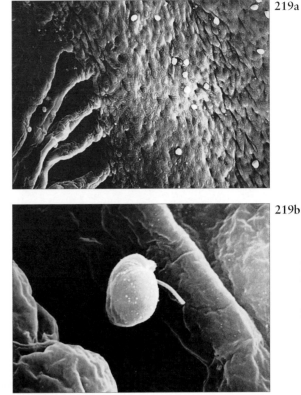

219a

219b

A gill biopsy of one fish reveals moderate numbers of *Ichthyobodo*. These scanning electron micrographs show *Ichthyobodo* on the gill of a fish (**219a**, ×200; **219b**, ×2,000). A skin scraping from the cloudy area along the dorsal body wall reveals very high numbers of the flagellate.
i. What is the treatment of choice for *Ichthyobodo* in the situation described?
ii. Are there other treatments that would be equally effective?

220 Suppose you are in a situation where you have diagnosed an ectoparasitic crustacean problem (e.g. fish lice, anchorworm) in a group of fish. The fish are sick and need immediate treatment. You are managing the water quality adequately and are ready to begin treatment. Name four parasiticide treatment regimens.

221 Where would you give an intramuscular injection in a fish?

219 **i.** A formalin bath (25 p.p.m.) applied directly to the display tank would be the easiest management strategy. Water quality parameters are appropriate and the owner should be reminded to maintain vigorous aeration during the treatment period. Water changes following the formalin bath are probably not necessary. One application of formalin should be adequate to control *Ichthyobodo*.
ii. Other treatment options include potassium permanganate, copper sulfate, and salt. Potassium permanganate could be used at 2 p.p.m. as a prolonged bath; however, it imparts a purple, then brown, color to the water. The discoloration of the water is highly undesirable in a display or exhibit tank. Therefore, potassium permanganate baths should usually be done in a treatment or quarantine tank. Copper sulfate is an excellent treatment for *Ichthyobodo*, but given the low alkalinity of the water (51 p.p.m.), it is contraindicated. Salt is also effective against many protozoal agents, including *Ichthyobodo*. Discus will tolerate only short-term salt treatments.

220 *Dimethyl phosphonate (trichlorfon):* 0.5 p.p.m., three treatments ten days apart, 20–30% water change 24–48 hours after each treatment. Use extreme caution when handling organophosphates. The liquid form commonly used to kill cattle grubs is easy to handle, measure, and dispense.
   Acetic acid: 2.0 p.p.m. as a 30-second dip is effective for treating new arrivals to a pond for crustacean parasites. Always test with one fish first, if possible.
   Dimilin: 0.01 p.p.m. for 48 hours, three treatments seven days apart. Very effective but this chitin synthesis inhibitor may kill desirable nontarget invertebrates.
   Saltwater/freshwater dips: may be effective against some parasites. Marine fish can be placed in a freshwater dip for 4–5 minutes and freshwater fish placed in salt water (35 p.p.t. salt) for 4–5 minutes.

221 Along the flank between the lateral line and the dorsal fin in most species. The needle is carefully inserted between the scales at about a 45° angle. Here we see a showa koi receiving an intramuscular injection (**238**).

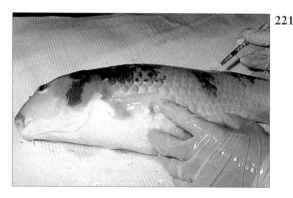

221

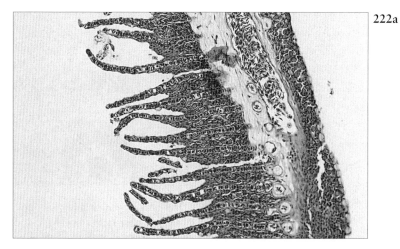

222a

222 i. Describe the lesion seen in this photomicrograph of a fish's gill (**222a**).
ii. What would normal gill tissue look like?

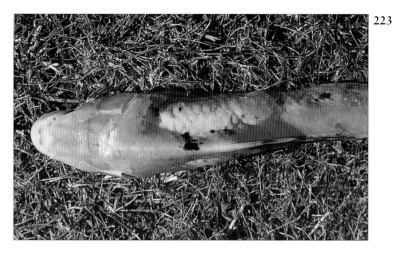

223

223 This is a photograph of a koi which had been suffering progressive weight loss for several months and was eventually destroyed humanely (**223**).

What procedures would you follow to carry out a histopathologic investigation into the cause of wasting in this fish?

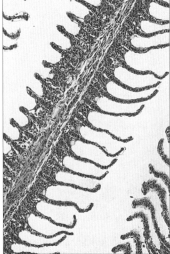

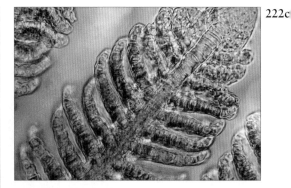

222 i. This is a section of a primary gill lamella with numerous secondary lamellae that are partially fused with one another. This is a case of secondary gill lamellar hyperplasia, probably due to an environmental toxin or bacterial pathogen.

ii. This histologic section is of normal healthy gill tissue (**222b**). Note the even, parallel, unfused secondary lamellae extending nearly perpendicular from the primary gill lamella. The fresh whole mount pictured here shows even secondary gill lamellae (**222c**). Note the lack of mucus or parasites.

223 Histopathology is one of the most useful and frequently used procedures in the investigation of fish disease.

Because postmortem degeneration occurs so rapidly in fish tissues, it is extremely important to obtain samples from fish that have been dead for no more than 30 minutes or from fish that have been sacrificed for examination.

Small pieces of tissue, no larger than a 0.5-cm cube, should be taken and placed immediately in an adequate volume of fixative (at least five times the volume of fixative to tissue). For general fish pathology, 10% neutral buffered formalin gives good tissue preservation.

Tissues sampled include the gill, skin (usually taken in the area of the lateral line and including a section of the underlying muscle), heart, liver, gut, spleen, and kidney. Other organs such as the eye, fins, or swim bladder, and brain may be sampled if appropriate and samples from any apparent abnormalities should also be obtained.

Samples should be submitted to an appropriate laboratory for histologic processing with an accompanying clinical history. Guidelines for the submission of pathology specimens should be followed closely.

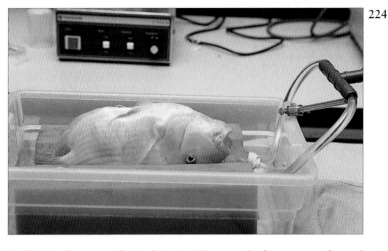

224

224 This fish has been anesthetized (**224**). What are the four stages of anesthesia in fish, and what would you observe during these stages when using tricaine methane-sulfonate?

225 A hobbyist client who raises a variety of killifish has been having a recurrent problem with mixed protozoal infections. You have helped her treat several out-breaks, each apparently caused by a different mixture of organisms. She shows her fish regularly and cannot pass up new and exciting specimens she finds at the shows. You have encouraged her to set up strict quarantine procedures, but she is reluctant to keep her short-lived new fish isolated for a prolonged period. Instead, she has decided that she wants to install an ozonation chamber on her main system, which recycles water through 50 tanks containing a total of approximately 5,000 L. Unfortunately, there are dozens of different ozonation systems, all touting different strengths and amounts, but all of the literature refers to bacterial infections. She has come to you for advice. What will you tell her?

224 Stage 1 Analgesia. This is observed as coordinated excitatory behavior with increased respiratory rate. This often appears to be a short stage of anesthesia in a fish that is induced with water-borne anesthetic agents such as MS-222. It is often difficult to determine where stage 1 ends and stage 2 begins.

Stage 2 Excitement. This is recognized by violent thrashing and jumping. A loss of coordination accompanies these behaviors. It is important to prevent the fish from injuring itself or jumping from its container during this time. Eventually the thrashing will subside, the fish will lose its equilibrium, and fin movements will cease. Reflex motion and response to tactile stimuli are maintained.

Stage 3 Surgical. Divided into four planes:

- Plane 1. The fish no longer responds to tactile stimulation. Respiration remains strong and the fish will respond to painful stimuli.
- Plane 2. Respiratory rate slows and there is a loss of response to painful stimuli. This is the most desirable depth of anesthesia for surgical procedures.
- Plane 3. Respiration is severely depressed.
- Plane 4. Further respiratory depression. Careful observation is required to observe any gill movement. Surgical planes 3 and 4 may be required for procedures requiring absolutely no movement. These procedures should only be attempted by persons experienced in fish anesthesia.

Stage 4 Cardiovascular collapse. All gill movements cease. Hypoxia may become evident as blanching of color from the fins. Death follows shortly.

225 Ozonation is becoming more popular for dedicated hobbyists with multiple tank systems. They should be advised of the risk of ozone to human lungs and encouraged to use systems that have a sealed contact chamber. Ozone can cause permanent lung scarring at levels that cannot be detected by the human nose. Your client should also be made aware of the effects of ozone on plastic and rubber. Systems must be checked frequently for deterioration of polymer parts. The contact chamber or countercurrent system should provide for a minimum of five minutes contact time and preferably ten minutes. This will reduce the risk of free ozone reaching the tanks. Attempts to solve problems caused by organisms that colonize tanks by ozonating side streams of water are rarely successful. Only the organisms that reach the contact chamber are affected by the ozone. Protozoa are less susceptible to ozone than most bacteria and require a higher dose. Your client should try to deliver approximately 90 $W/cm\ s^{-1}$ dose to the water through the ozone contact chamber.

226 i. Describe the lesion seen, and comment on how it may have developed (**226**).
ii. What is the most probable group of organisms associated with this condition?

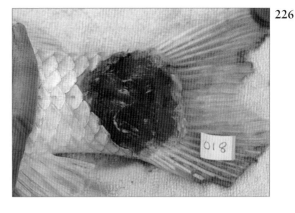

226

227 This red pacu was severely ravaged by a tank-mate and when found had bilateral deep ulcerative lesions which coalesced at the lateral midline of the fish (**227a**). Skin scraping revealed numerous *Tetrahymena* as well as some fungal hyphae consistent with *Saprolegnia*.

Knowing that pacu are very hardy fish, how would you manage this problem?

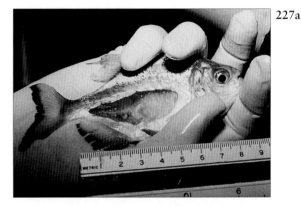

227a

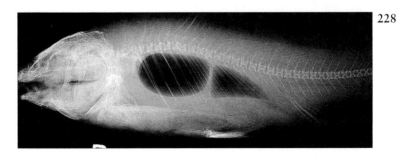

228

228 This is a lateral radiographic view of a butterfly koi (**228**).
i. Is the radiolucent swim bladder normal?
ii. How do koi and related fish regulate air in the swim bladder?

226 i. The photograph shows a large ulcer of the body wall of a koi carp with total sloughing of the skin and exposure of the underlying musculature. Such lesions can result from infection of superficial wounds, but are more commonly a sequela to generalized septicemia. Secondary infection by opportunistic bacteria or fungi commonly occurs and this may make the results of culture from the surface of such lesions confusing. When presented with a freshly dead fish, culture from the kidney may be more rewarding. Underlying stress factors such as poor water quality or chronic parasitism may contribute to disease development.

ii. A number of bacteria are associated with this condition, but the most common are the Gram-negative rods *Aeromonas* and *Pseudomonas*.

Some bacteria, however, are more pathogenic. Carp erythrodermatitis (also called 'goldfish ulcer disease') is caused by *Aeromonas salmonicida achromogenes*, a variant of the bacterium that causes furunculosis in salmonids. The organism is an obligate pathogen, although carriers can exist. It is relatively slow growing and fastidious, which can make it difficult to isolate from lesions.

227 The protozoal and fungal infections are secondary to the trauma sustained during the fish fight. You should be concerned about secondary bacterial infection and a loss of osmotic equilibrium in addition to the parasite and fungal problems. Daily saltwater dips (35 p.p.t. for 5 minutes) combined with an antibiotic in the

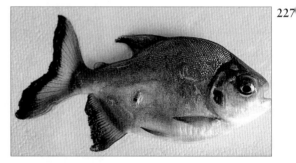
227

water (nitrofurazone at 20 p.p.m in this case) for 5–7 days would be an acceptable course of treatment. This particular fish responded well to the treatment and survived, although a permanent scar remains. This picture was taken three months after the trauma (**227b**).

228 i. This is the swim bladder of a normal koi. Koi, goldfish, and other cyprinids possess a swim bladder with two compartments.

ii. Koi, goldfish, and many fish without spiny fin rays (e.g. salmonids, characins) are physostomous, which means that they regulate gases in the swim bladder by a patent pneumatic duct that connects the swim bladder to the esophagus. Catfish, carp, and some eels possess both a patent pneumatic duct and a rete mirabile for gas regulation.

229 As a small animal practitioner in a metropolitan area, you have been offering clinical advice to local fish stores and occasional clients that own tropical fish. You have been seeing two or three pet fish clients per week, sometimes more. Recently, you have been seeing cases for advanced hobbyists who raise speciality fish for sale. Their problems and those of other clients sometimes are difficult to deal with on an outpatient basis. A logical step is to set up a small fish hospital ward. You have limited space, but you want to do a good job. You want to invest less than US$1,000 in the ward initially. Most of the cases you have seen have been small live-bearers and larger cichlids with infectious diseases (bacterial, protozoal, and fungal). The infectious diseases often seem to be secondary to husbandry problems. You would also like to be able to hold fish for surgical procedures.

What considerations should you include in your fish hospital ward design?

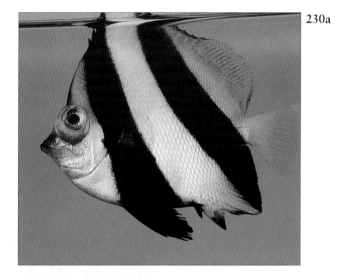

230a

230 This Moorish idol is markedly exophthalmic and on close inspection a large air bubble can be seen behind the globe (**230a**).
i. What is this condition called?
ii. How does this problem develop?
iii. How is this condition treated?
iv. List four other general causes of exophthalmia in fish.

229 Two important issues in a metropolitan area are water and air quality. The air you will bubble through the hospital tanks can concentrate chemicals normally found in low levels in veterinary hospitals. The air pumps you use should be located away from surgery, pharmacy, and kennel areas where potentially toxic anesthetics, disinfectants, and chemicals are used. It may be a good investment to put an activated charcoal filter on the intake of the air pump if you cannot provide a safe source of air. Metropolitan water sources must also be prefiltered or treated to be safe for fish. Activated carbon canister filters are adequate for the task, but you must be careful to change the media frequently. Exchange resin–fiber disc filters are a bit more expensive but it is usually easier to determine when to change the media based on the visible color changes. It is better to have several tanks rather than a single large one. Ideally, tanks should be independent and isolated from each other, but this is rarely feasible with limited space. You should rely primarily on water changes to maintain water quality, or use inexpensive sponge biofilters, so that disinfection between patients is relatively simple. Substrate which is required by some species should be limited to items that can be discarded or disinfected. Small tropical ornamentals do well in 20–40-L tanks. Your interest in surgical procedures will most probably result in you seeing larger individuals, so you will want one tank that holds at least 100 L. Control of tank temperatures can be handled economically by adjusting the ambient air temperature of the room where you keep the tanks if it can be warmed separately from the rest of the hospital. If not, or if you are seeing nontropical fish in addition to tropicals, you may need to use individual aquarium heaters. This requires multiple electrical outlets. Do not skimp on the electrical supply to your fish ward. Ground (earth) fault outlets are an important safety item. Submersible heaters are usually easier to disinfect than partially submersible units.

230 i. Supersaturation or gas-bubble disease.

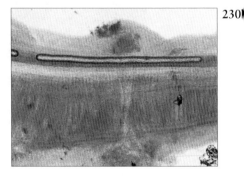

230b

ii. The most common cause of this problem is a cavitating pump which literally supersaturates the water with atmospheric air (meaning the majority of the gas will be nitrogen). Excessive oxygen production by algae and other plants is a less frequent cause. Over-aerating an aquarium with air bubbles from an air stone can, but rarely does, lead to supersaturation disease.

iii. Treatment usually involves finding the source of the excessive gas and eliminating it. In the case of a cavitating pump, filling the sump or reservoir or locating a leak in the system usually solves the problem. Air bubbles under the skin and within the fins will usually resolve within a day or two. Air bubbles in the circulatory system, especially in the branchial vasculature, can be acutely fatal (**230b**).

iv. Ammonia toxicity, ocular parasites, septicemia, and neoplasia.

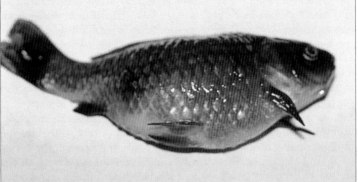

231 i. What clinical signs are visible in the figure (231), and what might one expect to see at necropsy?
ii. What are the main differentials, and what further tests would be necessary to confirm the diagnosis?

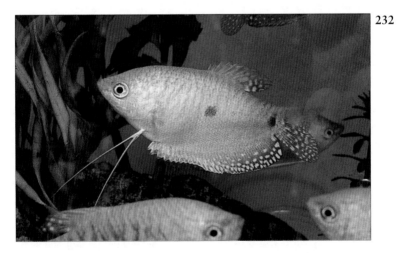

232 A local breeder you consult for has begun to experience mortalities in a few of her large vats of blue gouramis (232). Several in each vat have begun to darken and hang at the surface. You notice that a few have 'dropsy.' Water quality is fine.
i. What do you do?
ii. Should the breeder worry about the health of her gold gouramis, opaline gouramis, and platinum gouramis?
iii. How do you suggest that she manage this problem?

231 i. The photograph shows a goldfish with widespread hyperemia of the body surface and injection of the blood vessels of the fins. The abdomen is slightly swollen. These signs are nonspecific and are associated with generalized septicemia, toxemia, or viremia. Other signs may also be evident such as exophthalmos and more obvious abdominal swelling with raised scales.

At necropsy, one might see generalized erythema and hemorrhages of the visceral surfaces. Serosanguinous fluid may be in the abdomen. Peracute septicemias and viremias may occur in which there is mortality without prior clinical signs.

ii. The differential diagnoses include a wide range of bacterial, viral, and toxic agents. A careful history and examination of the environment might yield some important clues, but the definitive diagnosis is likely to be made at necropsy. The optimum site for bacterial sampling is posterior kidney. Smears should be stained with Gram and Ziehl–Neelsen stains and the appropriate media chosen for culture. A selection of samples of the major organs (heart, liver, spleen, bowel, kidney, gill, and skin/muscle) should be taken for histopathology.

Special precautions should be taken if the history is consistent with the possibility of spring viremia of carp (SVC) infection. In the UK, this disease is 'notifiable' and requires specific samples to be sent to the approved Ministry of Agriculture and Fisheries Laboratory for diagnosis confirmation. If a positive diagnosis is made, the Ministry has the power to impose restriction orders on the premises.

232 i. Sacrifice a few fish from each vat, perform complete external and internal necropsies, and take cultures of the kidney, liver, and brain, saving tissues for histopathology. Results: no external parasites are seen. Internally, many of the affected fish have clear amber fluid in their coelomic cavity and the intestines look hemorrhagic. Histopathology of the spleen reveals diffuse necrosis. Some of the fish sampled had bacterial infections, but over 50% did not. You send out sections of kidney, intestine, and spleen for virology. Results: positive for iridovirus.

ii. Yes, because all are color morphs of the same species. The virus appears to be a viscerotropic iridovirus which affects members of the *Trichogaster* genus, primarily *Trichogaster trichopterus,* but possibly *Trichogaster leeri,* the pearl gourami.

iii. This disease is currently not very well characterized. Predisposing factors may include overcrowding, poor water quality, and other stresses. Epidemiology of the disease is not well understood. Remove visibly affected fish, reduce stocking densities, and keep water quality excellent. Also use a disinfectant on utensils (nets etc.) between vats, disinfect vats when empty, and better still, keep separate equipment for unaffected fish. If possible, quarantine affected fish in an enclosed, separate area.

233 Two out of five tomtates being held in a quarantine facility were examined because of flaring of the gills and opercula (233). The affected fish appeared to have an increased respiratory effort compared with the unaffected fish. The fish were acquired two days before the onset of their illness. The other three fish appeared normal. The affected fish were lethargic and not eating. One of the affected fish was unable to orient itself in the water column.

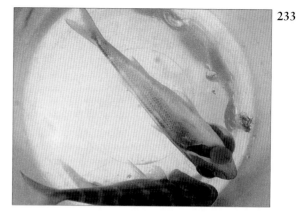
233

i. What are the possible causes of the clinical signs observed in these fish?
ii. How would you evaluate these fish?
iii. What are the possible causes of soft-tissue masses in the branchial arches of fish?
iv. What would your recommendations be for the remainder of the tomtates?

234 This clown triggerfish has presented for cachexia and inability to gain weight (234). The fish lives in an 800-L marine aquarium with a dozen other reef fish. The fish is eating a commercially prepared frozen marine fish food as well as some marine flake food. The other fish in the tank also eat this food. The owner is concerned that the fish has liver disease secondary to being captured with the aid of cyanide (the owner has no evidence to

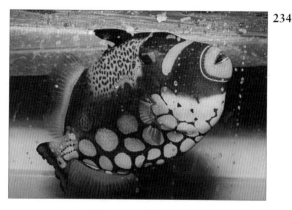
234

support this claim). Water quality parameters are within normal limits.
i. What will be your diagnostic plan?
ii. How will you manage this problem?

235 What is a safe volume of blood to remove from a fish for diagnostic or research sampling? How can this amount be determined?

233 i. Flaring of the gills and opercula of fish is suggestive of a respiratory disorder. Low levels of oxygen or toxic substances in the water may cause such signs; however, all the fish in the aquarium would be expected to show similar signs. Gill parasites, anemia, or masses in the area of the gills could also result in the clinical signs observed.
ii. A physical examination should be conducted with emphasis on the gills. If indicated, gill biopsies should be performed and examined for the presence of parasites and to assess the structure of the gill filaments. Upon physical examination of the affected fish, it was noted that both fish exhibited bilateral soft-tissue masses within the branchial arches. The affected fish died shortly after handling.
iii. The possible causes for the masses observed include thyroid hyperplasia (goiter), abscess, and neoplasia. Histologic evaluation of the soft-tissue masses revealed hyperplasia of thyroid tissue, indicative of goiter.
iv. The remainder of the tomtates, although clinically normal, were given an iodine supplement in a gelatin food at a dosage of 1 mg potassium iodide per kilogram of diet. Because these fish were recently acquired by the aquarium and there was no information available concerning their previous history, the goiters in the two affected fish may have resulted from a previous iodine deficiency; they apparently arrived with the condition. Another possible cause would include exposure to goitrogenic substances in the food or water before arrival.

234 i. In addition to a careful history, a complete diagnostic plan should include a fecal examination, radiographs, and blood tests. The serum chemistry values show no gross abnormalities (although reference ranges do not exist in this species) and the radiographs are unremarkable. A direct fecal examination reveals the presence of digenean trematode eggs. The fish weighs 200 g.
ii. There are two identifiable problems with this case. Although the fish is eating, you are not sure if the fish is getting enough food. A trematode infection is the second problem. In this case, the fish was given an intraperitoneal injection of praziquantel (6 mg/kg) and the fish was isolated and fed between 5% and 7% of its body weight per day of a balanced gelatinized food diet. Subsequent fecal examination was negative for parasitic ova and the fish steadily gained weight and body mass. Six months after treatment, the fish weighed 250 g and was strong, healthy, and in normal body condition. Because both the parasite treatment and the diet correction were applied at the same time, one cannot be sure which management practice contributed most to the fish improvement. It is likely that both problems had some effect on the fish.

235 Very little work has been done in the area of total circulating blood volume in fish. The tremendous number and variety of species contributes to this problem. A generally safe guideline is to assume that at least 3% of a fish's total body weight is blood and removing 10% of a fish's blood volume is safe for the animal. This means that a 100-g fish would have at least 3.0 ml of blood and it would be safe to remove 0.3 ml. Many fish species probably have total blood volumes in the 5–7% body weight range.

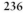

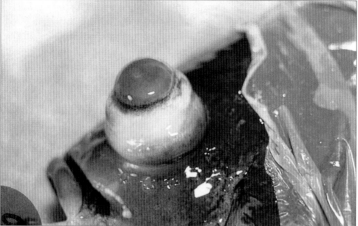

236 This oscar was exhibiting behavioral changes that the owner attributed to the eye lesion (**236**). What would be the probable cause and what procedures might be performed to confirm the diagnosis in the live fish?

237 Neighbors have recently moved to your area. They are experienced aquarists and have a freshwater tropical tank containing a variety of goldfish. Filtration in the tank is minimal and they have added an aquarium heater since the move. They are feeding their fish daily. The water is cloudy and the fish are sluggish. Some fish have died and a postmortem examination reveals gill epithelial damage with some lamellar hyperplasia. Your neighbors have moved from a water source with a pH of 6.5 into your area, which has more alkaline water (pH = 7.5). A water test reveals the following parameters:

Total ammonia nitrogen = 2.5 p.p.m.
pH = 7.5
Temperature = 20°C (68°F)
Un-ionized ammonia (1.6% of total ammonia nitrogen) = 0.04 p.p.m.

i. Why has the problem occurred?
ii. How can the situation be resolved?

236 The photograph shows an oscar with a swollen and protruding left eye. The condition developed gradually over a six-week period and the owner noticed behavioral changes in the fish, such as erratic swimming and banging its face on the side of the tank or other objects within the aquarium.

The protrusion of the eye was thought to be the result of a retrobulbar mass. The mass could possibly have been a tumor, abscess, granuloma, or localized edematous tissue.

The fish was anesthetized using benzocaine and the eye examined. Much of the cornea was opaque as a result of edema and there was hemorrhage into the anterior chamber. These changes made further ophthalmic examination impossible.

The prognosis was assessed to be guarded, and the eye removed surgically. Minor hemorrhage was controlled by pressure and the socket packed with a polybasic cream. Histopathology revealed multiple retrobulbar granulomata containing acid-fast organisms. Bacteriological isolation confirmed the presence of acid-fast organisms. Specific identification of the agent was inconclusive but was thought to be *Nocardia* rather than a mycobacterium.

Following surgery, the fish appeared well for a month. It then stopped eating and died soon afterwards. The owner wished to bury the fish in the garden and so necropsy was not possible. Similar granulomata were probably present in other body tissues.

237 i. The problem centers around the level of un-ionized ammonia in the tank.

Ammonia produced by fish as a waste product can shift between the ionized and un-ionized (toxic) form according to changes in water temperature and pH. The ionized form of ammonia is not too toxic to fish since they can excrete it readily through their gills and kidneys. The new neighbor has inadvertently increased the water temperature and the pH of the water for his fish tank.

When total ammonia nitrogen is measured, the total amount of nitrogen as both ionized and un-ionized ammonia is recorded. It is important to remember to calculate the percentage of un-ionized ammonia using the total ammonia nitrogen value. Tables are normally supplied with test kits that enable you to calculate the percentage of the total ammonia nitrogen that is present as un-ionized ammonia at a particular pH and temperature. Different fish species have different tolerances for un-ionized ammonia, but as a general rule of thumb it should not rise above 0.02 p.p.m.

ii. The situation can be resolved by gradually reducing the water temperature and reducing feeding (to reduce the amount of ammonia in the system); a reduction of stocking density should also be considered. More aeration, improved filtration, and regular partial water changes will all help to bring water quality back to healthy levels.

238 Which culture media are commonly employed in the isolation of bacterial pathogens of fish?

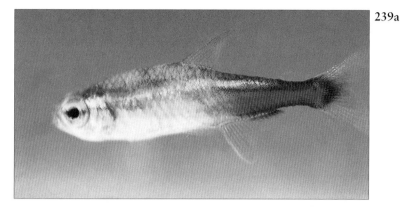

239a

239 This is a neon tetra from a community tank (**239a**).
i. What is your diagnosis?
ii. How would you treat this disease?

240 Three ultraviolet sterilizers are evident adjacent to a wet/dry trickle filter (**240**).
i. Is ultraviolet light treatment of water useful in preventing fish disease?
ii. How does an ultraviolet sterilizer work, and what are some factors that must be considered in order to maintain its effectiveness?

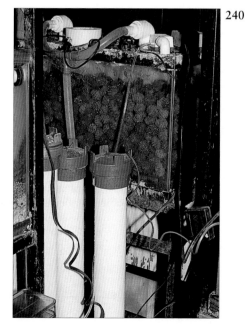

240

238 Many of the bacterial pathogens of fish are aerobic, Gram-negative rods which grow well on nonselective media such as tryptone soya agar. Bacteria, such as *Aeromonas*, *Pseudomonas*, *Pasteurella*, and *Vibrio*, may all be cultured on tryptone soya agar, although some marine organisms, including some *Vibrio*, may require supplementation of salt in the medium. Brain–heart infusion agar is an acceptable alternative to tryptone soya agar. For the isolation of mycobacteria, a special medium such as Lowenstein–Jensen agar is required. Generally, an incubation temperature of between 22°C (71.6°F) and 25°C (77°F) is appropriate for most ornamental fish pathogens. For the isolation of mycobacteria or *Nocardia*, a prolonged incubation period of several weeks may be required.

239 i. Neon tetra disease, caused by the microsporidian *Pleistophora hyphessobryconis*. This parasite infects muscle fibers causing wasting and focal color loss. In heavy infections, the disease may spread to the connective tissue of the intestine, ovary or skin. Diagnosis is made by identifying the characteristic spores, which are present in 'packets' (sporophorous vesicles) (**239b**).

ii. There is no proven treatment for any microsporidian parasite. A toltrazuril bath (20 p.p.m. for 1 hour every other day three times) has shown experimental efficacy against the vegetative stages, but not the spores, of another microsporidian, *Glugea*. The best method of control is destruction of infected stocks and disinfection of facilities.

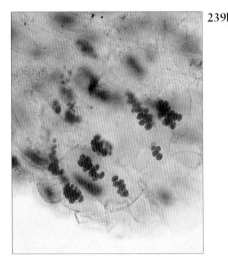
239b

240 i. Yes. Ultraviolet (UV) light sterilization of aquarium water is very helpful under the right conditions.

ii. UV sterilizers consist of a UV light bulb housed within a quartz tube allowing water to freely flow around the UV light source. UV light inactivates viruses, bacteria, protozoal parasites, and a variety of pathogenic spores by disorienting the structure of cellular DNA. For UV sterilization to be effective, enough energy must be delivered to kill the largest of the biological targets such as protozoans and the eggs of trematodes and other helminths. It has been determined that 180 microwatts per square centimeter is needed to kill *Ichthyophthirius*. To remain efficient and effective, UV systems require prefiltered water, a clean quartz tube, periodic tube replacement, and a sufficient number/size of bulbs to obtain the required energy level.

241 What precautions should you take to ensure a fish's well-being during an anesthetic procedure?

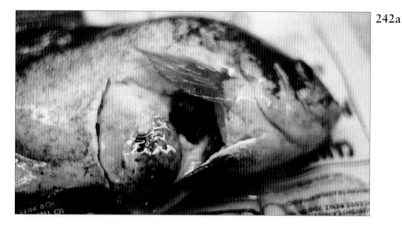

242a

242 This nine-year-old oscar had been anorexic and depressed for three weeks before dying. The owner reported that despite its reduced appetite during the preceding months, the fish 'continued to grow in the abdominal area.'
i. Based on the history and gross necropsy (**242a**), what is at the top of your differential list?
ii. How would you confirm the diagnosis?

243 This is a recently imported stick catfish (**243a**). There is a parasite visible near the oral cavity of this fish.
i. What is at the top of your differential list, and how would you confirm your diagnosis?
ii. Is this a common problem in aquarium fish?
iii. What are the clinical concerns with this condition?
iv. How would you treat this problem?

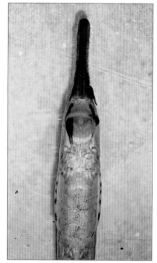

243a

241 The best way to avoid complications is by careful planning and the development of contingencies in case of a problem. The following list of precautions is far from exhaustive, but contains the important considerations:

- Double-check all anesthetic doses and calculations.
- Ensure adequate quality of water with the anesthesic.
- Provide supplemental aeration or oxygenation when appropriate.
- Keep the body, fins, and eyes of the fish moist during the procedure.
- Maintain adequate water flow over the gills.
- Have anesthetic agents available to deepen the plane of anesthesia if necessary.
- Have some means available to revive the patient if necessary.
- Transport of the patient should be minimized.

242 i. Neoplasia.
ii. Perform a complete necropsy and submit tissue samples in 10% formalin for histopathologic examination. In this case, the large, dark, sanguinous, fluid-filled mass in the caudoventral abdomen is part of the trunk kidney. The histologic section shows a single glomerulus and numerous abnormal papillary projections into the mesonephric duct (**242b**). This tumor was a mesonephric duct adenoma.

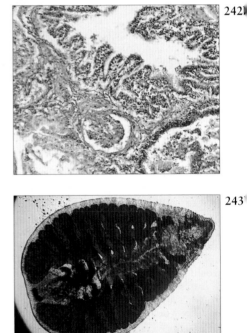
242b

243 i. The parasite is a leech or hirudinean. Low-power magnification confirms the presence of an anterior and posterior sucker, characteristics unique to leeches (**243b**). Digenean trematodes have an anterior and ventral sucker. Leeches are annelids and most are externally segmented.
ii. Leeches are uncommon in aquarium fish because they are relatively large parasites that are easy to remove. Most are detected and removed by tropical fish wholesalers and transhippers.
iii. Leeches can act as vectors for a variety of viral, bacterial, and parasitic diseases, as well as causing a mild to moderate anemia.
iv. If the fish can be caught, the leeches should be manually removed and disposed of. In a pond or larger aquarium, the organophosphate trichlorfon has proven to be effective.

244 The owner of a small ornamental pond has stocked *Plecostomus* for algae control. The pond has a heavy accumulation of detritus and the owner has been unable to clean the pond thoroughly for some time. The 15,200-L pond is designed to fit into a natural setting, and is in an area with many trees. Leaf debris, decaying plants, uneaten food, and fecal waste litter the pond bottom. The *Plecostomus* have recently developed small red ulcers on their peduncles. None have died, but a few appear weak and lethargic. Water quality parameters are shown below:

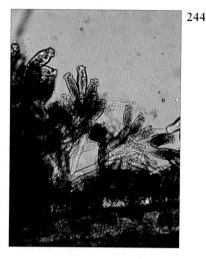

Dissolved oxygen: 5 p.p.m.
Chloride: 10.0 p.p.m.
Temperature: 28°C (82.4°F)
Total alkalinity: 256 p.p.m.
Total ammonia nitrogen: 3.1 p.p.m.
Total hardness: 220 p.p.m.
Nitrite: 0.3 p.p.m.
pH: 7.2

Skin biopsy of affected areas reveals mats of the stalked protozoan, *Heteropolaria* (**244**).
i. What is the most likely cause of the lesions observed on the fish?
ii. Which problem has the greatest potential to develop into a life-threatening situation, and why?
iii. What type of management or treatment strategy would be appropriate to correct the situation?

245 A goldfish pond owner contacts you and complains that although her goldfish appear fine, some minnows she had added to the pond have begun to die in large numbers. She claims her water quality is good and mentions the fact that a month ago she added three dozen minnows to the pond that she purchased from a local bait shop. The fish pic-

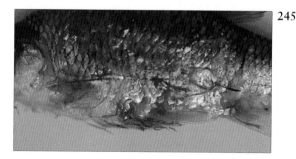

tured here was brought to you for inspection (**245**).
i. What is at the top of your differential list?
ii. What will your diagnostic work-up consist of?
iii. How will you treat this problem?
iv. What preventive medicine recommendations will you make?

244 i. The stalked, sessile protozoan, *Heteropolaria*, is commonly associated with red ulcerated lesions on fish. The parasite has a predilection for bony prominences and often is first evident as a raised area on the tips of fin rays. *Plecostomus* are particularly susceptible to *Heteropolaria* because of their sedentary nature, and the presence of overlapping bony plates, particularly on the peduncule. This protozoan seems to flourish in organically rich environments.

ii. *Heteropolaria* alone may not cause enough damage to result in mortality of affected fish. However, tissue damage at the attachment site can predispose fish to bacterial disease. Secondary infection with *Aeromonas hydrophila* is a common sequela to *Heteropolaria*, and can result in significant mortality.

iii. The treatment of choice for *Heteropolaria* is salt. The low chloride content of the water (10 p.p.m.) indicates that no salt has been added to the pond. For many ornamental ponds, a permanent application of 2.0 p.p.t. salt to the pond will control external parasite problems including *Heteropolaria*. A thorough cleaning of the pond should be recommended to remove organic debris and help prevent re-infestation. If fish were dying from a secondary *Aeromonas* infection, antibiotic use would be indicated. Bacterial culture and sensitivity testing should determine the correct antibiotic to use. Because these fish are housed in a 15,200-L pond, a medicated feed is the best method for delivering antibiotics.

245 i. An anchorworm (*Lernaea*) infection.
ii. The diagnostic work-up will consist of:

- A thorough history.
- Complete water quality test.
- Skin, fins, and gill biopsies.

iii. Once a pond is infected, the only way to get rid of the parasites, aside from draining the pond and removing the fish, is to treat the water with an organophosphate or a chitin synthesis inhibitor. If practical, infected fish may be caught and the parasites carefully removed with a pair of forceps or tweezers.

iv. Like most crustaceans, *Lernaea* lays eggs and these hatch into a microscopic, free-swimming larval form which eventually finds a fish and completes its life cycle as a parasite on the skin of the host. The eggs are located in paired sacs on the large female. Male anchorworms are microscopic. Fish infected with the early life stages will look normal. The best way to prevent this condition is to quarantine all new fish for at least six weeks and monitor them closely for signs of ectoparasitic disease. If quarantine is not possible, new fish may be dipped in salt water (35 g/L) for 3–5 minutes in an effort to kill larval stages. This dip will usually kill the adult parasites as well as the developing stages. Clients should be advised not to add bait fish to their ornamental fish ponds.

246 This butterfly koi presented for slight asymmetry visible in the trunk area at the level of the cranial aspect of the dorsal fin (246a). The fish was behaving normally but the owner wanted to know the source of the asymmetry.
i. What types of problems are on your differential list?
ii. What noninvasive diagnostic technique would you use?
iii. What vitamin deficiency may lead to this condition?

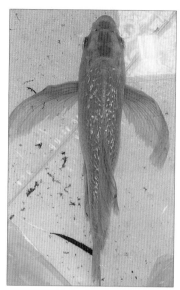

246a

247 i. What particular problem do freshwater fish face with regard to their osmoregulation?
ii. What physiologic mechanisms are in place to address this problem?

248 This group of firefish is clinically healthy (248). List two reasons why this statement can be made.

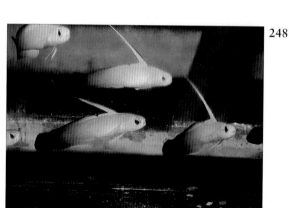

248

246b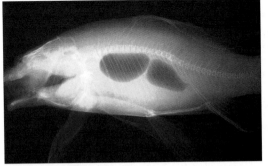

246c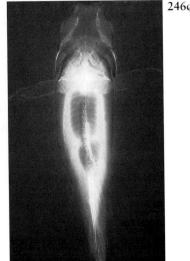

246 i. Scoliosis, neoplasia, ascites, and abscess or infection.

ii. Radiography. The spinal defect is difficult to see in the lateral view (**246b**) but evident in the dorso-ventral image (**246c**). This condition appears to be common in koi and may be nutritional, genetic, or traumatic in origin. Affected fish may remain stable or the condition may progress.

iii. Vitamin C.

247 i. Freshwater fish live in an environment in which their body fluids are hypertonic to the surrounding water. As a result of diffusion and osmosis, there is is a tendency for water to enter the fish's body and for salts to leave it. It is essential for the normal physiological processes of the fish that the concentrations of the body fluids are controlled within narrow limits.

ii. The regulation of body fluid concentrations in freshwater fish is achieved by three principal factors:

- Limitation of the overall permeable surface area. The skin with its mucus layer ensures that the skin surface remains impermeable. Thus the surface area available for the exchange of water is reduced to that of the gill, and to a lesser extent the bowel. This factor is important in those diseases in which the skin surface becomes ulcerated.
- Excretory processes within the kidney. Freshwater fish produce a large volume of very dilute urine, aided by the efficient resorption of sodium and chloride ions from the kidney tubules.
- Excretory processes in the gill. Active and passive transport mechanisms within the acidophil cells of the gill allow for the exchange of sodium for hydrogen and chloride for bicarbonate.

248 This species of schooling fish is swimming as a group. Erect dorsal fins, bright colors, clear eyes, and even fin margins are evident.

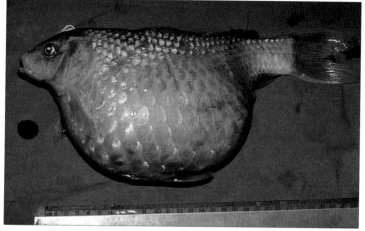

249

249 i. What abnormal clinical sign is shown in this photograph (**249**)?
ii. What are the possible causes, and what is your diagnosis?

250 A local dairy farmer has decided to build an ornamental pond. He has the advantage of using clear fresh water pumped from a deep borehole on his land. The water is used all over his farm and appears to be of good quality. He has never kept fish on this site before.

The construction of the pond is satisfactory and filtration appears adequate. The only unusual feature of the pond is its shape. Because of the space available, the farmer has a circular pond measuring 2.0 m in depth and 0.8 m in diameter. He has used a new black PVC fruit storage barrel as the pond liner. Plants have been placed around the edge of the pond. Six koi (0.2 m in length) were placed in the pond. No aeration or filtration was put in the pond. Within 24 hours, all the fish have died. There were no external signs of disease; however, two out of the six fish showed some degree of exophthalmia. Samples of pond water brought to you for testing show that all parameters are within normal limits.
i. What is your probable diagnosis?
ii. How would you confirm this?

249 i. The photograph shows a carp with a grossly distended abdomen. The swelling is symmetrical and upon palpation appears to be filled with fluid.
ii. The swelling could be due to a number of factors:

- Free fluid within the abdominal cavity.
- Tumor, cyst, or granuloma within the abdominal cavity.
- Tumor, cyst, or granuloma within the body wall.

Lesions within the body wall generally appear as asymmetrical swellings and so can usually be distinguished upon clinical examination. The same is the case for intra-abdominal masses, although it is possible that these could cause a secondary build-up of fluid and hence be difficult to distinguish from ascites. Free fluid can accumulate following any disruption of fluid balance (renal or gill disease), and may also be a sequela to myocardial damage produced as a result of a toxemia or septicemia. A specific diagnosis may be difficult to make in the live fish. Ultrasonographic evaluation as well as aspiration of the fluid might be valuable. Exploratory laparotomy may also be warranted. The definitive diagnosis is often only made at necropsy.

250 i. The farmer seems to be doing everything right apart from choosing to have a pond with a relatively small surface area and not using aeration and filtration. However, with only six fish in the pond, he should not to have to worry about water quality. The clue should be in his choice of using deep borehole water. If every water quality parameter when tested off site appears normal and the client is using borehole water, be suspicious of gas supersaturation. Most probably, the problems are connected with carbon dioxide or nitrogen. Another clue is the exophthalmia noted in two out of the six fish. When water has become supersaturated, small bubbles are often seen in the fins of the fish between the fin rays or around the loose connective tissue of the eye (hence the signs of exophthalmia). If gas supersaturation were a problem, the relatively small surface area of the pond would not help to eliminate the gas from the water. The depth of the pond (without movement of water by filtration and aeration) will also slow down elimination of carbon dioxide or nitrogen from the water.
ii. The best way to prove the diagnosis is to take samples of water straight from the borehole into airtight jars, completely filling them with water. The sample should be taken from the borehole pipe itself. Measurement of gases in water can be problematic in the general testing situation. Regional laboratories responsible for checking drinkable water quality will be helpful in either performing the test for you or letting you know who can do this test. A pH test on site may help to identify the problem.

A quick comparison should be made of the pH of this water compared with well-aerated water collected from the pond. If carbon dioxide supersaturation is the problem, the borehole water will have a lower pH.

The problem is due to pressure differences. As the water reaches the surface, gases that are normally under pressure and in solution below ground come out of solution at the surface, where only 1 atm (101 kPa) of pressure exists (rather like opening a carbonated soft drink for the first time). In this particular case, carbon dioxide supersaturation was diagnosed as the problem.

251 How might the problem in 250 be prevented?

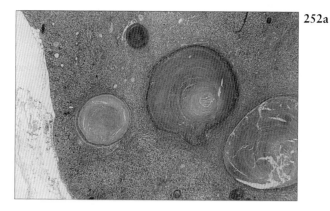

252a

252 Histopathologic examination of tissues from the fish in the previous question revealed the presence of multifocal granulomata throughout several organs (252a).
i. What is your presumptive diagnosis?
ii. What differential staining procedures could be used to verify your diagnosis?

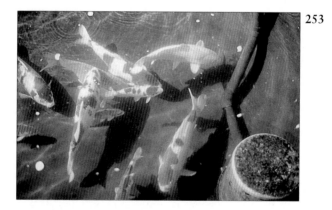

253

253 The owner of an ornamental backyard pond, located in a heavily wooded neighborhood, has observed night herons near his pond at dusk. Occasionally, the birds have been observed removing fish. The pond owner is frustrated because valuable fish have been taken, often within one to three days of being placed in the pond (253).
i. Based upon the narrative provided, what is your initial assessment of the situation?
ii. What changes in management could be made to alleviate the problem?

251 The pond water should be aerated and a filtration system installed. Attempts to prevent layering or stratification of the water should be made using a submersible pump circulating water from the bottom of the pond and spraying it onto the surface. It is difficult for some pumps to lift water by 2 m, so the client must be sure to have a powerful pump. Care should be taken each time the pond is topped-up with borehole water to ensure that the supersaturation problem has been solved.

252 i. Granulomatous diseases are fairly common in ornamental fish. Causative agents include mycobacteria and *Nocardia* (frequently grouped together as 'piscine tuberculosis') and systemic fungal infection.
ii. Differential staining of the histologic sections may help in determining the precise cause of the disease. Mycobacteria are generally acid-fast when stained using the Ziehl–Neelsen technique. *Nocardia* are weakly acid fast. Although both mycobacteria and

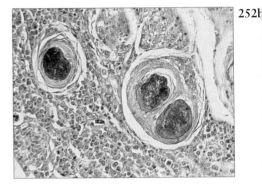

252b

Nocardia are Gram-positive, it is very difficult to demonstrate this characteristic (**252b**). Fungi may be demonstrated using a silver-impregnation technique such as the Grocott method or by using the periodic acid–Schiff reaction; however, the fungus may have been destroyed by the inflammatory response and no causative agent may be visible.

253 i. Brightly colored fish, particularly when swimming near the surface, are extremely attractive to piscivorous birds. Birds will frequently roost in trees near the affected pond and quickly develop a habit of visiting the pond when hunting.
ii. Pond design can be used as a deterrent to predation. Steep sides with depth greater than 45–60 cm makes it difficult for some wading birds, such as the night heron, to catch fish. Pond cover with plants, such as broad leaf water lilies, will provide some protection from hunting birds. Covering the pond with bird netting, shade cloth, or screening is very effective in the elimination of bird predation; however, cost and esthetic concerns should be addressed. A number of devices are marketed as bird deterrents. These include scarecrow-type objects, artificial birds of prey, and brightly colored streamers. Birds may become accustomed to these objects over time. Audible deterrents are also available including propane cannons, recordings of distress calls, calls of birds of prey, and various computer-generated sounds. It may be necessary to reconsider the species of pond fish appropriate for stocking. Brightly colored fish may be impossible to maintain in this situation unless the pond is heavily planted or covered. Alternative species might include fish indigenous to the area, suggesting a more natural setting.

254 An ornamental fish pond in a garden has been in operation for five years with no previous problems. It is heavily stocked with goldfish, tench, rudd, and a few large koi. There has been a recent period of hot, dry weather. Consequently, the water temperature is 5°C (9°F) warmer than usual. The water has turned green. The pond has a filtration system and aeration is supplied as a trickle of water circulating continuously, entering one corner of the pond.

Early one morning, the owner finds that 25% of his largest fish are dead. The remaining fish are crowding at the surface of the water near to where the trickle of water enters the pond.
i. Why did the fish die?
ii. What is your immediate advice?
iii. What long-term advice can you give to prevent recurrence of the problem?

255a

255 A moderately stocked 75-L community tank has been running for three months with no significant problems. Filtration and heating are adequate, and weekly 20% water changes are made. An incandescent hood containing two 40-W full-spectrum bulbs was added three weeks ago (**255a**). For the past two weeks, the owner has complained of recurrent 'Ich' problems (presumptive) despite multiple treatments with a commercial malachite/formalin product.

All water parameters are within normal limits with the exception of the temperature, which is 30°C (86°F).
i. What is the likely cause of disease in this system?
ii. How would you correct the problem?

254 i. The whole picture is one of low dissolved oxygen in the pond. The fish that died were asphyxiated. In hot weather, when the water temperature rises, the solubility of dissolved oxygen in water is lower. Phytoplankton thrive in sunny conditions; they remove carbon dioxide from the water and produce oxygen by photosynthesis, but they remove oxygen from the water at night as the respiration pathway takes place. With high feeding rates (and the fish would initially feed very well at higher water temperatures), more feces and waste enters the pond. Various bacteria break down this food (using up more oxygen). The amount of oxygen in the water will vary throughout the day. It will be lowest in the early morning before photosynthesis begins again. The fish are showing signs of oxygen deficiency by crowding around the area in the pond where there is likely to be the highest oxygen concentration.

ii. This is an emergency situation. Remember that the surviving fish will be severely stressed. The immediate recommendation is to provide adequate aeration. This can be done by agitating the surface of the water or attaching a spray device to the aeration equipment. Allow the water to spray up in the air to strip oxygen from the atmosphere before dropping back into the pond. Feeding should be severely reduced. It would be best to feed a few small meals in early- to mid-afternoon when photosynthesis is at its peak. Aeration should be continued throughout the night until the crisis is over. A dissolved oxygen meter would be very beneficial.

iii. The long-term advice is based on explaining how oxygen depletion has killed his fish. The owner should be advised to assess the stocking density of the pond and be aware of the consequences of overstocking. After the problem has passed and the fish have returned to a normal, unstressed state, the pond should be cleaned out and water quality tests carried out on a regular basis. Cleaning out the pond will remove a lot of organic matter which consumes oxygen. It would be a good idea to have additional aeration equipment and a holding tank available in the future so that the fish could be split between the pond and the additional tank, thus reducing stocking density and improving oxygenation for the fish.

255 i. The high-wattage incandescent lights being used in this system are likely to transfer too much heat to the water. Daily elevations of the temperature constitutes a chronic stress, which may immunosuppress the fish and predispose them to opportunistic infections.

ii. To correct the situation, the owner may change to two 20-W incandescent

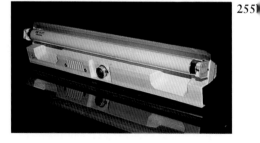

255b

bulbs, or if a higher degree of illumination is desired, to a fluorescent light source (255b), which transfers significantly less heat to the aquarium water. It is unlikely the fish truly had 'Ich' as this parasite does not thrive at 30°C (86°F).

256 You are presented with a problem in which all the fish in a garden pond are suddenly found dead.
i. What would be your provisional list of differentials?
ii. How would you go about investigating the problem?

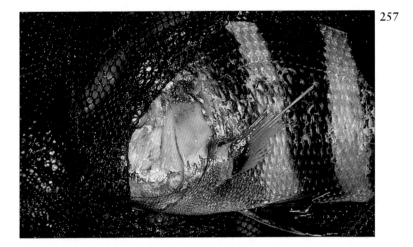

257

257 This sheepshead was presented with a necrotic cutaneous lesion on the left side of its head (**257**). It was housed in an outdoor concrete pool with several other marine fish, including other sheepsheads. The fish was being slowly acclimated to freshwater by dropping the salinity by 0.5 p.p.t. per day. The salinity was 2.5 p.p.t. when this fish was presented for evaluation. The water temperature was 24°C (75.2°F) and maintained by a submersible heater that was added to the pool to provide additional heat during cold weather.
i. What are the possible causes for the cutaneous lesion, and how can they be differentiated?
ii. How would you treat the lesion in this fish?
iii. How could this condition have been prevented?

256 i. The possible differential diagnoses are:

- Exposure to a toxin.
- An environmental factor causing a sudden drop in dissolved oxygen.
- A peracute viral or bacterial infection.

An infection is very improbable as even the most virulent organism is unlikely to result in a sudden 100% death rate. An examination of the environment and measuring the routine water quality parameters (including dissolved oxygen) will be of value in discounting a sudden drop in dissolved oxygen.

If a toxin is suspected, the investigation should proceed with caution and accurate records kept as it may develop into a case of litigation. The history may give a possible clue as to the source of the toxin, and it is worth contacting the local water authority to inquire if the problem is widespread.

ii. The possible avenues of investigation are:

- Necropsy of the fish. If fresh material is submitted, a full necropsy including sampling for bacteriology and histopathology should be performed. Such investigations should confirm a peracute infection.
- Samples for toxicology should be taken at this time in case the bacteriology is negative or the histopathology is suggestive of such a problem. Paired tissue samples of liver, muscle, and brain should be collected and frozen.
- Water samples for toxicology. Paired samples of at least one liter of water should be collected in inert containers filled to the top so as to exclude air. If the samples need to be stored, they are best filtered and kept frozen.

257 i. Possible causes for the cutaneous lesion observed on the side of the head of the sheepshead would include traumatic injury, bacterial infection, parasitic infestation, or mycotic infection. A scraping from the lesion might reveal the presence of an etiologic agent when examined on a wet mount or stained smear. In this case, the wet mount and stained smear failed to demonstrate protozoa or other etiologic agents. It was determined that this fish liked to hide behind the exposed heating element that was added to the pool. Therefore, the lesion most probably resulted from a burn on the left side of the head.

ii. The fish was isolated by placing it in a floating mesh basket that prevented contact with other fish. A topical antibiotic ointment containing a corticosteroid anti-inflammatory agent was applied to the wound twice daily. After 30 days, the lesion had healed completely and the fish was released from the basket back into the pool.

iii. Exposed heating elements should be enclosed in a protective covering that will prevent contact with fish. The burn patient may have been using the heater as a hiding place or was seeking warmer temperatures.

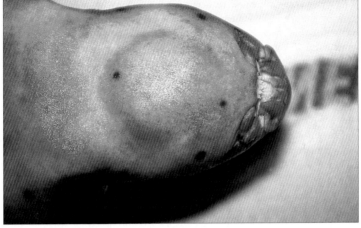

258

258 A small horn shark presented with a large, round, soft-tissue swelling in the area of the throat (258).
i. What are the possible causes of the lesion?
ii. How can a quick presumptive or definitive diagnosis be made?
iii. How would you treat for goiters in a shark?

259 i. What organism can be identified in this photomicrograph (259)?
ii. With what clinical signs might it be associated?
iii. What treatments are commonly recommended for its control?

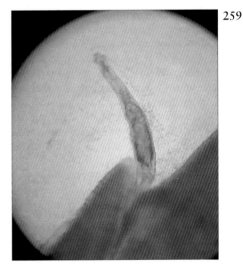

259

258 i. The most common cause of a large, round, soft-tissue swelling in the ventral throat area of sharks is thyroid hyperplasia or goiter. Other possible causes would include inflammatory disorders, such as granulomatous lesions, and neoplasia.
ii. An aspiration biopsy of the tissue for cytologic evaluation can be helpful in differentiating between inflammation, neoplasia, and tissue hyperplasia. In this case, an aspiration biopsy revealed a poorly cellular sample that contained occasional uniform-appearing epithelial cells. A presumptive diagnosis of thyroid hyperplasia was made based upon the lack of evidence of inflammation or neoplasia and the appearance of epithelial cells suggestive of tissue hyperplasia.
iii. An iodine supplement is the treatment of choice for goiter in sharks. Potassium iodide was given biweekly at a dosage of 10 mg/kg. After two months, the mass had decreased greatly in size and nearly disappeared. All the sharks in the system were supplemented with 250 mg calcium iodate in tablet form per kilogram of food fed. This type of supplement is easy to provide to large sharks but difficult to provide to smaller sharks. An alternative to oral supplementation would be to add iodine to the aquarium water allowing the sharks to absorb the iodine either through the gills or when they ingest the aquarium water. Heavy oral supplementation of iodine in the food of sharks in a closed system will elevate the iodine concentration in the sea-water and will aid in the prevention of goiter.

259 i. The photomicrograph is of a gill squash preparation under low power. A single gill fluke (*Dactylogyrus*) is attached to the gill lamellae. Careful examination of the parasite as it moves free of the gill tissue will reveal the presence of eye spots and the absence of paired hooks which are characteristic of *Gyrodactylus*.
ii. In moderate numbers these flukes can cause significant gill irritation resulting in excessive mucus production and gill hyperplasia.
   Grossly, the gills appear swollen and have a grayish color, caused by the mucus covering the surface. The reduced oxygen uptake may cause an increased rate of opercular movements and fish may gather at the surface of the water, below waterfalls, or near air stones.
iii. A number of treatments are commonly recommended for controlling monogenean flukes. Formaldehyde added to the water is often used. Organophosphorus is also used, but may not be available for use in all countries. Marine species respond well to reversed salinity.
   Dactylogyrus is an oviparous species so cleaning and disinfection of tanks may be useful to eliminate the eggs. The eggs are resistant to chemical treatments so repeated treatments may be necessary to control the problem.

260 You are brought a large paradise fish for examination. It is listless and lethargic. There are no specific external signs. The owner has had the fish for nearly ten years. It is the lone survivor of a mixed tank that her son kept when he was a teenager. When the son left for college six years ago, there were three or four fish left in the tank, and the mother has cared for the fish since then. A large 'algae eater' was the last fish to die, nearly a year ago. It followed the same pattern, slowly losing appetite and weight, and becoming listless. It was then found dead on the bottom one morning. The owner was not aware that veterinarians saw fish at that time. She is attached to this fish, which comes to be fed each day.
i. What do you suspect?
ii. What would you do?

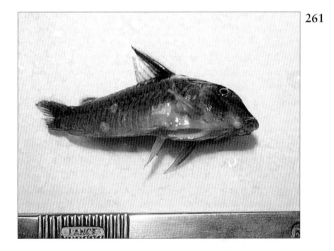

261

261 A client contacts you and is concerned that her cory catfish are sick. She recently purchased them from a pet store and placed the five fish in her 200-L community aquarium. Like the fish pictured here, all five had distinct, pale white to yellow, subcutaneous nodules visible in all areas of the body (261). The fish were behaving normally and the rest of the fish in her tank were fine. The owner did not notice the nodules in the pet store but remembers seeing them shortly after introducing the fish to her well-lit aquarium.
i. What are these nodules?
ii. How can you confirm your diagnosis?
iii. What is the life cycle of this parasite?
iv. Can or should this condition be treated?

260 i. A very common problem in long-established tanks that begin to show unexplained mortalities is improper water changes leading to accumulation of salts and toxins from feed and aeration. The lack of specific external signs supports this diagnosis.

ii. The first step would be to perform routine water analysis. A high ammonia level could be the result of transporting the fish in the water, and would not be expected with this history. High nitrates or copper levels would be more probable and would not be caused by transport. In extreme cases, water conductivity can be increased by the accumulation of salts.

Impression smears and gill biopsies can be performed to rule out common infectious diseases, but these are unlikely as a primary problem in a fish that has been isolated for a year. It would be wise to avoid further stressing the fish. Instruct the owner in the proper method for performing a water change. Many people are unaware of the difference between changing water (when water is removed and then replaced to the same level) and topping off (when water is added to return the tank to normal levels replacing evaporation losses). Have the owner perform a 50% water change every other day after instructing her on proper conditioning of replacement water. Be sure to caution her to avoid temperature shock. Fish suffering from multiple toxicities because of chronic stale water usually respond rapidly, regaining their appetite and vigor within days.

261 i. These nodules represent the encysted metacercaria of a digenetic trematode, most likely belonging to the genus *Clinostomum*. This condition is common in wild-caught or pond-raised cory catfish, Australian rainbowfish, and pond-reared live bearers such as guppies, mollies, and platys. Aquarists and aquaculturists frequently call this condition yellow or white 'grub' disease.

ii. Using a scalpel, forceps, and fine scissors, the metacercaria can be teased from its cyst and examined under the microscope. The presence of an oral and ventral sucker confirm its identity as a digenean trematode.

iii. The fish is actually an intermediate host for this parasite. The definitive host is usually a fish-eating bird or other higher vertebrate, and a molluscan invertebrate, usually a snail, is the first intermediate host.

iv. This condition is usually not harmful to fish and cannot be transmitted to other fish in the aquarium without the definitive and first intermediate hosts being present. In severe cases where the metacercaria are very numerous or involve internal organs, clinical signs including general debilitation and weight loss can be observed. There is evidence that treatment using parasiticides that target trematodes (praziquantel, 5–10 p.p.m. for 24 hours as a bath immersion) will kill the metacercaria.

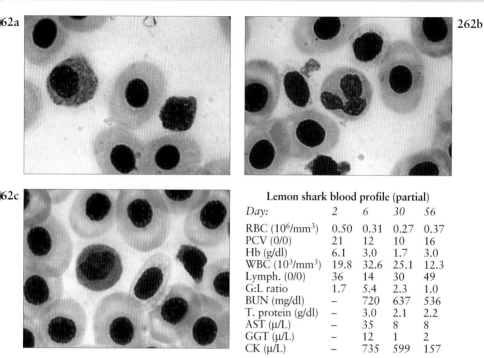

Lemon shark blood profile (partial)				
Day:	2	6	30	56
RBC (10^6/mm³)	0.50	0.31	0.27	0.37
PCV (0/0)	21	12	10	16
Hb (g/dl)	6.1	3.0	1.7	3.0
WBC (10^3/mm³)	19.8	32.6	25.1	12.3
Lymph. (0/0)	36	14	30	49
G:L ratio	1.7	5.4	2.3	1.0
BUN (mg/dl)	–	720	637	536
T. protein (g/dl)	–	3.0	2.1	2.2
AST (µ/L)	–	35	8	8
GGT (µ/L)	–	12	1	2
CK (µ/L)	–	735	599	157

262 A captive male lemon shark, measuring 44.1 kg in weight and 190 cm in length, had a two-day-old deep bite wound on the caudal one-third of his caudal fin. The deep wound involved the caudal vertebrae and was unstable. Blood was taken for a complete blood cell count (day 2). Four days later, the wound was observed to be filling with a red colored tissue. A blood sample was taken for a blood profile (day 6) and a systemic antibiotic (amikacin, 3.0 mg/kg intramuscularly every 72 hours) was initiated for a total of seven treatments. Twenty-four days after the initiation of the antibiotic therapy, the shark was evaluated and a third blood profile was obtained (day 30). The wound remained unstable and did not appear to be healing. The caudal tip of the tail did not appear viable and was surgically removed just cranial to the original bite wound. The tissue was allowed to granulate closed. After 26 days, the wound had nearly healed by establishment of a healthy granulation bed that was being covered by normal appearing epithelium. A fourth blood profile was obtained at this time (day 56).

i. What are the cells in the peripheral blood of this shark in figures **262a–c**?
ii. How would you assess the blood profile changes between days 2, 6, 30, and 56?

263 You are in a situation where you have diagnosed an internal nematode problem in a group of fish. The fish are sick and need immediate treatment. You are managing the water quality adequately and are ready to begin treatment.
  Name two parasiticide treatment regimens.

262 i. Lemon sharks have three types of granulocytes in the peripheral blood along with two types of mononuclear leukocytes, lymphocytes, and monocytes. They also have nucleated erythrocytes and thrombocytes. **262a** demonstrates a G1 granulocyte, a lymphocyte, and mature nucleated erythrocytes. The normal G1 granulocytes typically resemble avian heterophils except that they tend not to have a lobated nucleus. Normal G1 granulocytes have prominent round to oval eosinophilic cytoplasmic granules and a colorless cytoplasm. **262b** demonstrates a G2 granulocyte, two thrombocytes (adjacent to the G2 granulocyte), and mature nucleated erythrocytes. There is a small, mature lymphocyte with a scant amount of blue cytoplasm below the G2 granulocyte. The cytoplasm of the thrombocytes is colorless in contrast with the blue cytoplasm of the lymphocyte. The G2 granulocytes of sharks often have a lobed nucleus and a colorless cytoplasm (when stained with Wright's stain). They lack the distinct eosinophilic cytoplasmic granules observed in G1 and G3 granulocytes. **262c** demonstrates a G3 granulocyte, a thrombocyte, a lymphocyte, and mature nucleated erythrocytes. The G3 granulocyte of sharks resembles the avian eosinophil, except that they tend not to have a lobated nucleus. They have distinct eosinophilic cytoplasmic granules that are round and have tinctorial properties that differ from the G1 granulocytes. In general, G2 granulocytes have brighter eosinophilic granules and a blue cytoplasm when compared to G1 granulocytes. **262c** demonstrates the difference between a thrombocyte with a colorless cytoplasm and a lymphocyte with a blue cytoplasm.

ii. The changes in the erythron between day 2 and days 6 and 30 are suggestive of a blood loss anemia. The improvement in the red blood cell parameters on day 56 indicate that the shark is responding to his anemia. The leukogram changes reflect a leukocytosis with slight improvement between days 6 and 30. This could reflect a favorable response to the antibiotic therapy; however, a significant inflammatory response still exists on day 30. The granulocyte to lymphocyte (G:L) ratio shows a significant increase between day 2 and day 6. This, along with the increase in the total leukocyte count, is indicative of a severe inflammatory response. The improvement in the G:L ratio on day 30 supports a favorable response to therapy. The return of the G:L ratio to normal (1.0–1.5) by day 56 is a favorable sign. The blood biochemistries indicate high blood urea nitrogen (BUN) values typical of sharks. Sharks utilize urea nitrogen to maintain their normal plasma oncotic pressure. The significant changes in the biochemical profile include elevations in aspartate aminotransferase (AST), gamma glutamyltransferase (GGT), and creatine kinase (CK) enzymes on day 6 that show decreases on day 30 and a return to normal by day 56. This is suggestive of a recovery from severe skeletal muscle damage that resulted from the bite wound to the tail. Removal of the necrotic tissue helped return the blood profile to normal parameters.

263 *Fenbendazole:* combine in food at a concentration of 0.2% and feed for three days. Repeat in 14–21 days.

Levamisole: use as a bath treatment at a concentration of 2.0 p.p.m. for 12–24 hours and repeat in 14–21 days. Always test new drugs on a single fish first!

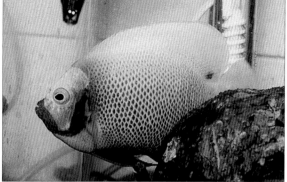

264

264 This marine angelfish has a chronic erosive lesion of the head around the eye (264). The entire area is depigmented and devoid of normal epidermis.
i. What is this condition called?
ii. What are some probable causes of this syndrome?
iii. How would you manage this problem?

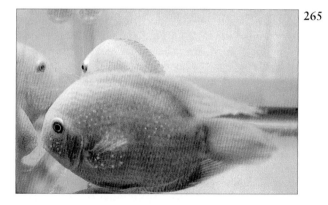

265

265 A pair of adult gold severums were purchased by a hobbyist for use as broodstock. They were placed in a 38-L aquarium equipped with a sponge filter and air stone. Water temperature was adjusted to 26°C (78.8°F). Seven days after arrival, the fish were lethargic and the owner noticed they were completely covered with white dots (265). He phoned the individual who had sold him the fish, a trusted friend, and was assured that the fish had never been sick during the 18 months they had been in his care. He had purchased them as juveniles from a reputable pet store and never had to question their health.
i. What is the most likely problem, and how would you confirm your diagnosis?
ii. What is the most probable source of the infection?
iii. How should the problem be managed?

264 i. Head and lateral line erosion (HLLE). This is a chronic condition associated with negligible mortality. Affected fish usually have been in captivity at least several months. Tangs (Acanthuridae) and marine angelfish (Pomacanthidae) frequently display lesions. Gross inspection may reveal small pits in the epidermis around the head and lateral line progressing to large, usually nonhemorrhagic ulcers. These lesions are frequently without pigmentation and may extend the length of the lateral line. The disease is usually nonfatal but can result in permanent scarring.

ii. The primary etiology of HLLE has not been discovered, although environmental stresses such as poor water quality, inadequate nutrition, and the presence of opportunistic pathogens appear to be involved. Recent reports of a reovirus isolated from a moribund angelfish displaying the initial lesions associated with HLLE may support the theory of an immunocompromised state existing in fish affected with HLLE.

iii. HLLE does not usually kill fish and affected individuals have been known to survive for years with only mild progression of clinical signs. For resolution of this condition, a change in husbandry is nearly always required. Improving nutrition combined with removing external stresses (aggressive tankmates, poor lighting, etc.) may arrest or even reverse the syndrome. Treatment with antimicrobials alone is unsuccessful; however, resolution of the lesions has been seen with vitamin-C supplementation or elimination of activated charcoal from the filtration systems.

265 i. White spots on fish can have several causes. However, the most common cause of white spots on freshwater ornamental fish is the ciliated protozoan parasite *Ichthyophthirius multifiliis*. Identification of *I. multifiliis* should be confirmed by taking a sample of skin mucus from an area exhibiting white spots, preparing a wet mount, and examining it with a light microscope.

ii. The affected fish were most probably carriers of the infection. Fish that survive infection by *I. multifiliis* retain some immunity to the organism, but may carry a small number of encysted parasites that emerge at a later time, frequently following a change (usually a decrease) in water temperature.

iii. Controlling *I. multifiliis* in a freshwater aquarium is relatively straightforward, and several approaches are possible. The first is simple chemical control, which implies application of an appropriate compound to the water, at a designated concentration for an appropriate period of time. Effective compounds include formalin (25 p.p.m. as an indefinite bath or 170–250 p.p.m. for 30–60 minutes), potassium permanganate (2 p.p.m. as an indefinite bath, or up to 10 p.p.m. for 30 minutes), copper sulfate (safe use is based on total alkalinity of the water), and salt (0.03% as an indefinite bath or 3% for up to 10 minutes – when the fish rolls over and appears stressed, move it to fresh water). A second strategy used to control *I. multifiliis* is temperature control. Tomites (juveniles) are not tolerant of water temperatures above 32°C (89.6°F). Raising water temperature to this level for five consecutive days is effective in elimination of emerging tomites from the aquarium.

A third strategy that can control *I. multifiliis* is careful cleaning of infested aquaria daily with particular attention paid to siphon particulate debris from the bottom and sides of the glass.

Index

Jack Dempsey 116
Jacknife fish 48
Jewel cichlid 136

Kanamycin 117
Ketamine hydrochloride 110
Kidney 53, 59, 85, 96, 121, 135, 148, 150, 180, 223, 231, 232, 242, 247
Killifish (*Nothobranchus* sp.) 184, 225
Koi 14, 30, 31, 33, 39, 41, 66, 69, 75, 83, 98, 105, 112, 134, 137, 143, 158, 159, 163, 168, 170, 182, 189, 204, 209, 213, 223, 228, 246, 250, 251, 254

Labyrinth organ 197
Laparotomy 249
Leech (hirudinean) 27, 139, 149, 243
Lenticular cataract 75
Leporinus fish 100
Lernaea sp. 149, 192, 205, 245
Lesser octopus 45
Leukocyte 108, 262
Levamisole 62, 141, 263
Lionfish 16, 123, 172
Liver 74, 223, 231, 232
Lordosis 199
Loricariid catfish 27
Lowenstein-Jensen agar 47, 238
Lymphocystis disease 48, 165
Lymphosarcoma 1

Malachite green 88, 113, 125, 255
Melanin 148, 198
Melanomacrophage center 23
Melanophore 4, 108
Mesonephric duct adenoma 242
Metronidazole 91, 118, 132, 142
Midas cichlid 36, 97
Mollies 12, 55, 191, 261
Molt-inhibiting hormone 5
Moorish idol 230
Muskellunge 1
Mycobacterium spp. (mycobacteria) 47, 64, 91, 92, 204, 238, 252

Neascus sp. 198
Neon tetra disease 13
New tank syndrome 114
Nitrite toxicity 117
Nitrifying bacteria 7, 120
Nitrofurazone 43, 124, 227
Nitrogen cycle 6, 7, 206
Nocardia spp. 47, 238, 252
Nuclear bone scan 31
Odontogenic hamartoma 3

Oil of cloves 69, 95
Oodiniasis 100
Operculum 20, 72, 89, 93, 155, 156, 158, 165, 208, 233
Orfe 100
Organophosphate/organophosphorus 8, 66, 211, 220, 243, 245, 259
Oscar 110, 132, 179, 236, 242
Osmoregulation 135, 247
Otoliths (ear stones) 150
Ovarian prolapse 14
Ovary 71
Oxygen 16
Ozonation 19, 63, 93, 225

Pacu 214, 227
Pancreas 74
Papilloma 33, 63, 77, 101
Paradise fish 260
Pasteurella spp. 238
Pearci chichlid 209
Pearl cichlid 91, 136
Pearl danio 169
Peduncle disease 30
Periodic acid-Schiff reaction 252
Perkinsus marinus 183
Pharyngeal pad (muscle) 26
Pharyngeal teeth 26, 34, 97, 150
Photosynthesis 254
Phytoplankton 254
Pictus (Pimelodus) catfish 57, 164, 186
'Pine cone' appearance 52, 70, 137
Planehead filefish 15
Platy 29, 44, 62, 151, 261
Plecostomus sp. 114, 116, 117, 136, 139, 244
Pleistophora sp. 13, 239
Pneumatic duct 36, 60, 68, 228
Popeye disease 52, 152, 191
Potassium iodide 233, 258
Potassium permanganate 160, 178, 191, 219, 265
Povidone iodine 69, 147
Praziquantel 141, 146, 198, 234, 261
Predation 157, 203, 253
Proecdysis 5
Pseudobranch 20, 152, 153
Pseudomonas spp. 40, 122, 226, 238
Pulse oximetry 9

Quarantine 2, 16, 43, 48, 90, 104, 107, 136, 139, 154, 176, 182, 200, 225, 232, 233, 245
Queensland grouper 72

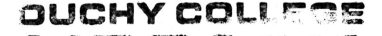